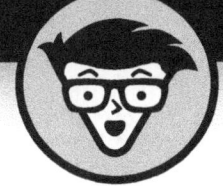

Weight-Loss Medications

by Patrick Reeves, MD, FAAP, DABOM and
Tania Elliott, MD, FAAAAI, FACAAI

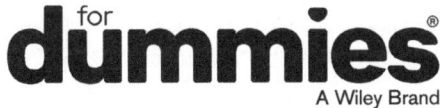

Weight-Loss Medications For Dummies®

Published by: **John Wiley & Sons, Inc.**, 111 River Street, Hoboken, NJ 07030-5774, www.wiley.com

For general information on our other products and services, please contact our Customer Care Department within the U.S. at 877-762-2974, outside the U.S. at 317-572-3993, or fax 317-572-4002. For technical support, please visit https://hub.wiley.com/community/support/dummies.

Wiley publishes in a variety of print and electronic formats and by print-on-demand. Some material included with standard print versions of this book may not be included in e-books or in print-on-demand. If this book refers to media such as a CD or DVD that is not included in the version you purchased, you may download this material at http://booksupport.wiley.com. For more information about Wiley products, visit www.wiley.com.

Library of Congress Control Number is available from the publisher.

ISBN 978-1-394-37522-6 (pbk); ISBN 978-1-394-37524-0 (ebk); ISBN 978-1-394-37523-3 (ebk)

Printed and bound by CPI Group (UK) Ltd, Croydon, CR0 4YY
C9781394375226_260126

Contents at a Glance

Table of Contents

Introduction

L osing weight today looks very different than it did a decade ago, and this book walks you through the tools that actually work. You can dive into details about modern weight-loss medications — the ones that can help people lose 15 to 22 percent of their body weight when used correctly. And you can see what the research really says about these treatments, including what happens when you stop them.

To help you best understand how doctors make decisions about your care, we explain the major obesity guidelines and give you a peek at the studies that show you why lifestyle changes still matter even when medications are part of your plan. And if you're looking for an alternative to medicine, we cover that, too, introducing you to the top choices, including bariatric surgery and endoscopic procedures, which remain the most powerful options for long-term weight loss.

Because weight loss is a holistic effort, we give you more information than just meds in this book. We explain how behavioral therapy, exercise, and nutrition patterns like the Mediterranean diet support steady progress. And we cut through the hype to help you understand what science actually reveals about the benefits of supplements like fiber, green tea extract, probiotics, and berberine. We also emphasize why ongoing care matters, including follow-up, coaching, and support, as well as help you select a care team.

Each option has strengths and limitations, and most people need more than one tool to reach their goals. Weight loss is not only about willpower but about biology, environment, and long-term strategy. We want you to feel more confident choosing the path that fits your life and your health, so you can use the information we've included in this book to understand the full menu of weight-loss options and select the kind of care and support you need.

About This Book

This book is here to help you understand weight loss in a clear, practical way. You will learn what the modern medications do, how they work, and how to use them safely. You will also see how lifestyle changes, nutrition, movement, and behavioral support fit into a real plan that lasts.

This book walks you through each major class of weight-loss medications and how doctors choose between them. You will also learn how to set up a care team, talk with your clinician, and understand the tests and screenings you may need. You will see how diet, exercise, and supplements can help these medications work better and how to adjust these tools for your age and health needs. We even account for special populations that have additional considerations when it comes to care. So if you want to understand more about the unique needs of women, older adults, children, and people with complex health conditions, this book covers it as well.

And because not everything ever goes as planned, you can also learn what to do when medications do not work the way you expected. This includes behavioral strategies, non-medication approaches, and the procedures that offer more weight loss than medicine alone. And we answer important questions surrounding weight loss, such as what the scientific studies say about long-term results, muscle preservation, and how to avoid weight regain, and we cover insurance issues, cost questions, and how to stay safe when using telehealth or online services.

This book is a reference book. So while we include all of the important topics you need to be successful and supported in your weight-loss journey. You don't have to read it cover to cover. Of course, we'd love for you to dive into every detail we've included, but consider this book a full map of all the tools available for weight loss. You will have the background to make informed decisions, ask better questions, and choose the path that fits your life. And most importantly, you will understand that weight loss is not about willpower. It is about using the right tools, at the right time, with the right support.

Foolish Assumptions

To best meet your needs and answer all your questions when writing this book, we made a few assumptions about you:

>> You're carrying extra weight, maybe even struggling with obesity, and you're ready for real help, not hype.

>> You're motivated to lose weight because you want to feel better, move easier, and live longer.

>> You want to lower your risk of serious health problems like diabetes, high blood pressure, heart disease, or liver disease.

>> You've heard about weight-loss medications but aren't sure how they work, if they're safe, or whether they're right for you.

>> You may be starting from scratch with no medical background, and you want clear explanations in plain language.

>> You're open to learning how medication, lifestyle change, and ongoing support can work together, not as a quick fix, but as a real plan.

Icons Used in This Book

We use icons in this book so you can quickly and easily identify specific information that you'll find useful:

REMEMBER

This icon highlights key takeaways to help you understand how weight-loss medications and GLP-RAs work and how they fit into your long-term health journey.

TIP

Look for this icon for practical advice you can use right away. This icon will highlight simple strategies you can use to get the most benefit from your medication and lifestyle changes.

WARNING

Pay close attention to these sections. They point out common pitfalls, safety concerns, or misconceptions that could interfere with your weight-loss journey. This icon also helps you steer clear of unsafe medication practices.

TECHNICAL STUFF

This icon signals a deeper dive into the science or medical details behind weight-loss medications and GLP-RAs. It's interesting and helpful for some readers, but you can skip it if you just want the essentials.

Beyond the Book

If you're looking for a quick, easy reference to the most important information in this book, be sure to check out the Cheat Sheet created just for you. You can find it on the Dummies website — go to www.dummies.com and search for the title of this book. The Cheat Sheet gives you a big-picture overview of weight-loss medications, including GLP-RAs, as well as important weight-loss information, all in one easy place. You can use the Cheat Sheet to access important information quickly and conveniently even when your book isn't handy.

Where to Go from Here

We've organized *Weight-Loss Medications For Dummies* into four sections:

>> Part 1 lays the foundation for everything that follows. This section introduces the world of weight-loss medications and explains why obesity is best understood — and treated — as a chronic medical condition rather than a personal failure. You'll learn how modern medications, including GLP-1 and GLP-1/GIP receptor agonists (GLP-RAs), were developed, how they work in your body, and why they've changed the landscape of obesity care. This part also helps you understand the differences between available medications, what makes one option a better fit than another, and what "responsible use" looks like from the very beginning. If you're new to weight-loss medications or want to better understand what you're taking and why, this is the place to start.

>> Part 2 focuses on what it looks like to use weight-loss medications safely, effectively, and in partnership with your healthcare team. You'll walk through what to expect at clinic visits, how clinicians screen for risks, and how decisions are made about starting, adjusting, or switching medications. If you want to know how to get the most benefit from your medication while protecting your health, Part 2 is your roadmap.

>> Part 3 tackles the real-world complexities of weight-loss treatment. Bodies, lives, and medical histories aren't one-size-fits-all — and this section reflects that reality. You'll learn how weight-loss medications are used across different ages, sexes, and health conditions, and how chronic illnesses like diabetes, heart disease, or fatty liver disease influence treatment plans.

>> Part 4 is designed for quick reference and practical comparison. Here you'll find curated top ten lists that summarize key takeaways from the book, including the most effective medications, influential research studies, and non-medication strategies that still make a meaningful difference. These lists are especially helpful when you want fast answers, side-by-side comparisons, or evidence-based talking points to bring to your healthcare visits. Think of this section as your shortcut to clarity when you don't have time to reread entire chapters.

You are probably really excited to dig in and figure out how best to start your own weight-loss journey, but we get it if you feel overwhelmed and aren't sure where to begin. You can begin reading anywhere you like, but we've given you some good starting points based on what you might be interested in most:

>> If you like to start at the beginning, go ahead and turn the page to Chapter 1. We'll walk through this together.

>> If weight-loss medications feel confusing or overwhelming, start with Part 1. It explains what these drugs actually do — and what they don't.

>> If you keep hearing about GLP-1s and aren't sure what applies to you, Chapter 2 breaks it down in plain language.

>> If you're asking yourself, "Is this safe?" or "Is this even right for me?", head to Chapter 3. These are honest answers, not hype.

>> If you already have a prescription in hand, Part 2 helps you use it well and avoid common mistakes.

>> If eating feels different, exercise feels harder, or side effects are getting in the way, Chapter 5 is for you.

>> If the scale has stopped moving, or you're worried that your excess weight will all come back, Chapter 6 talks about what's normal and what actually helps.

>> If your situation feels more complicated than most, turn to Part 3. Bodies and lives are not one-size-fits-all.

>> If medication hasn't worked the way you hoped, or you can't take it, Chapter 9 shows you other paths forward.

>> If you're thinking about surgery but feel unsure or nervous, start with Chapter 10. Knowledge makes decisions easier.

>> If you just want quick answers right now, flip to Part 4. Short lists. Clear comparisons. No fluff.

1

Getting the Scoop on Weight-Loss Medication

Get a clear introduction to the world of weight-loss medications, including how these drugs were developed, how they work, and why they have become such an important tool in treating obesity.

Understand the basics behind GLP-1 and GLP-1/GIP medications (GLP-RAs), the differences between available formulations, and what makes one medication a better fit than another.

Explore how these medicines influence appetite, fullness, metabolism, and long-term weight trends, and see what responsible use looks like from day one.

Chapter **1**

Tracing the Path of Weight-Loss Medications

Medications for weight loss have a long and sometimes wild history. People have been trying to manage their weight since ancient times. Early remedies included herbal laxatives and strange tonics that promised to melt fat but mostly caused discomfort. Some people even went as far as swallowing tapeworm eggs because they hoped the parasite would do the work for them. As time passed, we moved into an era of stimulants and appetite suppressants, and many of those drugs worked at first but carried risks we only understood later.

You might wonder why any of this matters when you are here looking for answers today. It matters because it shows that the struggle you feel is not new and it is not a personal failure. People have been searching for real solutions for centuries. History shows that people in your shoes often tried things that were unsafe because they were desperate for help. When you understand where we started, you can appreciate how far the science has come and why safety matters more than ever. You also see that you're not alone in this and that your desire for a healthier life connects you to many others who have walked this road. Today, we finally have options that focus on health rather than punishment and fear. Modern medications are built on decades of learning from the mistakes of the past. This chapter gives you the background you need so you can move forward with confidence and choose what is safe and effective for you.

Sifting through the Science: Early Experiments That Helped and Hurt

People have been trying to solve the challenge of weight for as long as we have written history — a powerful reminder that you are not alone in this. Even though the tools have changed, the same themes keep showing up as people search for answers, hope, and relief. Many treatments through the centuries promised breakthroughs but fell short because they were unsafe or misunderstood. However, each one of these therapy failures taught us something important about how the body really works. In this section you will see how those lessons shaped the medicines we have today. This illuminates the science behind current treatments and how these medicines give you a much stronger chance of having an effective weight-loss journey.

Ancient times through the 19th century: Looking for weight-loss answers

The pursuit of weight loss is as old as recorded medicine. Ancient Greek and Roman physicians, such as Hippocrates and Soranus of Ephesus, advised lifestyle changes like reduced food intake, avoidance of fullness, regular exercise, and sometimes nighttime running.

In addition, these ancient physicians recommended herbal mixtures which turned out to cause more harm than good. These treatments did not support health; they pushed the body into distress because people were desperate for any tool that might make them thinner. Hellebore, for example, was a powerful purgative that caused severe diarrhea, dehydration, dizziness, and, in higher doses, even heart problems or death. Scammony was another strong laxative resin that irritated the gut so intensely that people often developed cramping, electrolyte loss, and dangerous weakness afterward. Honey water seemed gentle, but when used in excess as a cleansing agent it could lead to fluid shifts and ongoing diarrhea that weakened the body. Cnidian berry was believed to "cleanse" the system, yet historical accounts describe nausea, vomiting, and intense abdominal pain after taking it. Even donkey milk with honey, which sounds mild today, was used in quantities that acted as a laxative and sometimes caused prolonged digestive upset.

TECHNICAL STUFF

If you're searching for what *not to do*, you can read more about these practices in several ancient medical texts. Much of this information appears in the writings of Hippocrates, particularly in works like *On Regimen* and *Airs, Waters, Places*. It is important that you keep in mind that these well-intentioned but failed ancient therapies are simply the stepping-off point to a safer weight-loss journey which you can take starting now.

REMEMBER

Up until the 19th century many physicians encouraged people to limit food intake, eat bulky foods (these were probably high in fiber), take baths before meals, and engage in hard exercise. Some of these ideas were reasonable because eating more fiber and moving your body can support health in many ways. These are still helpful habits, and you will see your doctor recommend them today. These simple lifestyle changes are now based on evidence and have been shown to help you feel full and keep your metabolism steady.

WARNING

Other practices were far less helpful and sometimes harmful because they were based on dangerous guesswork rather than science. Elixirs that contained opium, ginger, cinnamon, myrrh, saffron, and castor oil were used often, and some of these ingredients carried real risks. Opium caused sedation and addiction. Castor oil caused severe cramping. Myrrh and saffron caused digestive irritation. Some physicians even tried harsh tactics like stitching a person's mouth partly shut so that they could only take liquids. These measures were signs of how desperate people felt to control their weight. Those practices are not supported in today's state-of-the-art medical field.

This history matters because it shows why safety must come first when you explore treatment options today. Many older drugs were pulled from the market after scientists discovered how dangerous they were. Your doctor now uses evidence, lab testing, and close follow-up to help you find a treatment that supports your health. Some people start with lifestyle changes and then add medications slowly to see how they respond. Others may have health conditions that make GLP-1 medicines a good place to begin. A good doctor helps you make this decision together and guides you through the safest and most effective plan for your body.

1930s to1950s: Relying on research

The 20th century brought an explosion of research into weight loss, and new medications began appearing faster than ever before. Scientists were learning more about metabolism, appetite, and hormones, and many of these discoveries led to drugs that promised real hope. But once medications reached the public, researchers often found that some did not work as expected and others carried risks that only became clear after years of use. This is why post-release research is so important — it helps us see which treatments truly help people and which ones need to be removed to protect patient safety. For example, several weight-loss drugs have been pulled from the U.S. market after serious health concerns came to light:

>> Fenfluramine, which became widely used in the 1970s and later paired with phentermine as Fen Phen, was withdrawn in 1997 after it was linked to dangerous heart valve damage.

» Sibutramine was approved in 1997 and stayed on the market until 2010, when studies showed a higher risk of heart attacks and strokes.

» Ephedra, a stimulant found in many herbal weight-loss products in the 1990s, was banned in 2004 because it raised blood pressure and caused life threatening heart rhythm problems.

These drugs often looked promising when they first came out, but real-world use revealed risks that outweighed their benefits. You will read more about these drugs and others in the later section, "Suppressing appetites in the 1960s to 1970s." The stories of these medical therapies for weight loss remind you why strict testing, careful monitoring, and a good doctor by your side matter so much when you start any modern weight-loss treatment.

New medications from this time period include

» **Thyroid hormone:** When doctors first began experimenting with thyroid hormone for weight loss, it marked a major shift in how medicine approached obesity. Until then most treatments relied on herbs, purging, or extreme lifestyle rules, and none of them were based on real science. As physicians learned more about how the thyroid controls metabolism, they noticed that people with overactive thyroid glands tended to be very thin. This sparked the idea that boosting thyroid hormone might help people lose weight in a more predictable way. It felt like an exciting leap forward because it was one of the first times doctors used a biological explanation instead of guesswork. But even though the logic made sense, the results were risky. You would not want this treatment today because it caused muscle loss, heart-rhythm problems, tremors, diarrhea, and in some cases life-threatening complications. Because of these dangers, your doctor should not prescribe thyroid hormone for weight loss unless you have an actual thyroid disorder that needs treatment. This chapter shows you how these early scientific attempts shaped the safer, more targeted options you have today.

» **Dinitrophenol (DNP):** In 1933, researchers discovered that DNP, a chemical previously used for explosives, could dramatically increase weight loss by stimulating energy production in cells and speeding up metabolism. Weight came off quickly, but users suffered overheating, cataracts, peripheral neuropathy, and, in many cases, death. By 1938, the FDA banned DNP in one of its earliest safety-driven drug withdrawals.

DNP is still found on the black market. Its use for weight loss is illegal and potentially fatal.

» **Amphetamines:** First synthesized in the late 1800s, amphetamines started to be used in the 1930s as appetite suppressants. By 1937, generic and branded amphetamines were widely prescribed for weight loss. Amphetamines changed chemicals in the brain called norepinephrine and dopamine, which made people feel alert and less hungry.

TECHNICAL STUFF

Dopamine is mainly produced in two regions deep in the brain: the substantia nigra and the ventral tegmental area, both part of the midbrain. Its true job is to help regulate movement, motivation, learning, and the feeling of reward. When dopamine works the way it should, it helps you stay focused, enjoy pleasurable experiences, and learn from them. Norepinephrine is produced mostly in a small structure in the brainstem called the locus coeruleus. This chemical helps control alertness, attention, stress response, and the fight or flight system. When norepinephrine rises, your brain becomes sharper and more awake, which is why stimulants can make you feel energized but also jittery or anxious.

WARNING

You may recognize these names because they also affect mood and focus. When amphetamines force these chemicals to rise too high, you may feel a burst of energy at first, but your body eventually pays the price with crashes, mood changes, and dependence. Over time doctors learned that these pills caused addiction, high blood pressure, severe insomnia, and personality changes. Because of these risks, you should not be given amphetamines for weight loss today. Your doctor may prescribe them for attention disorders, but that is a very different medical use which requires strict monitoring.

The stimulants from weight-loss history remind you that not every fast-acting treatment is a safe one. Further, it shows why you deserve a doctor who guides you toward options with real evidence and real safety checks (see Chapter 4 for more on putting together a health care team).

1960s to 1970s: Suppressing appetites

These decades marked a major turning point in weight-loss medicine because researchers were beginning to understand the brain's role in appetite and metabolism. New medications came to the market that felt more modern and more targeted, and many people were hopeful that safer options had finally arrived. At the same time, this period exposed how quickly things could go wrong when drugs were released without strong long-term safety data. In this section you will see how promising ideas, risky experiments, and new regulations all shaped the weight-loss landscape that your doctor works within today.

>> **Phentermine:** Phentermine was approved in 1959 and is still prescribed today, which makes it the longest standing weight-loss medication you might actually be offered. Doctors liked it in the 1960s and 1970s because it was less intense than classic amphetamines and seemed to curb appetite without the same level of addiction risk. Phentermine works by stimulating the release of norepinephrine in your brain, which signals your body to feel less hungry. It

also slightly increases your energy level, so you may feel more alert while eating less. It did become a mainstay during that time, and some people still use it today under close medical supervision. You should know that phentermine is still a stimulant, so it can cause palpitations, insomnia, anxiety, and increased heart rate. These risks are not ancient history. They still matter for you now, and your doctor will monitor you closely if this is part of your plan.

>> **Fenfluramine:** Fenfluramine hit the U.S. market in 1973, offering appetite suppression by enhancing serotonin release in the brain. Initially, doctors saw it as a promising alternative to stimulants. However, the combination of fenfluramine and phentermine (later known as "Fen-Phen") would become the most high-profile, and ultimately notorious, weight-loss regimen in history (see the later section, "Exploring the Fen-Phen era," for more details on this drug).

>> **The rainbow pills:** The rainbow pill craze took off in the 1960s and early 1970s, and it remains one of the most chaotic and dangerous chapters in weight-loss history. These packs contained mixtures of amphetamines, barbiturates, thyroid hormone, diuretics, and laxatives, and each pill had a different effect on your body. The amphetamines suppressed appetite by boosting dopamine and norepinephrine, while the barbiturates sedated you so you did not feel overstimulated. Thyroid hormone ramped up your metabolism, and the diuretics and laxatives forced rapid water and stool loss that looked like weight loss but was not real or safe. If you had walked into a clinic then, you might have been handed a rainbow packet with no explanation of what each pill did. These combos led to addiction, heart attacks, psychiatric events, and deaths, which triggered Senate hearings and tighter FDA action in 1967 and 1968. Because of these changes, you will not see anything like rainbow pills prescribed today. Their history is a powerful reminder that fast weight loss is never worth risking your life, and it shows why you deserve safe, evidence-based care with a doctor who truly understands this landscape.

1990s: Exploring the Fen-Phen era

Combining phentermine with fenfluramine (or dexfenfluramine), Fen-Phen produced rapid, significant weight loss and soared in popularity throughout the 1990s. At its peak, millions took it, often for months or years. But soon, severe side effects emerged — most notably heart valve damage and primary pulmonary hypertension, conditions often fatal or requiring surgery. By 1997, the FDA requested withdrawal of fenfluramine and dexfenfluramine, ending the Fen-Phen chapter and re-emphasizing the need for long-term safety data.

REMEMBER

Only phentermine remains available today under close monitoring.

UNCOVERING THE FAILINGS OF FEN-PHEN

Fen-Phen became one of the most talked about weight-loss treatments in the 1990s, and for a while it seemed like everyone knew someone who was taking it. The combination came together because phentermine was already FDA approved in 1959 and fenfluramine was FDA approved in 1973. Doctors began prescribing them together even though the FDA had never formally approved the two drugs as a single combined therapy. At the time this was allowed because physicians could legally prescribe approved drugs "off label," and many believed the pair worked better than either drug alone. This created a buzz that spread through weight-loss clinics, and demand grew very fast.

People taking Fen-Phen often lost weight quickly, but the excitement did not last. As more patients used it, doctors started to see serious heart valve problems that were hard to ignore. These cases kept showing up, and eventually researchers connected the issue to fenfluramine.

In 1997 the FDA withdrew fenfluramine from the market, and the era of Fen-Phen came to an abrupt end. This withdrawal pushed regulators to strengthen safety monitoring after drugs reach the market, and it led to stricter rules for tracking rare but serious side effects. The Fen-Phen story reminds you why early enthusiasm can never replace good science and why you need a doctor who puts your safety above fast results. It also set the stage for the much more careful testing standards that guide today's weight-loss medications, including the newer GLP-RA treatments.

2000s: Prescribing safer pills due to stricter standards

The 2000s brought a new wave of weight-loss medications that entered the market under much stricter safety standards than in earlier decades. Regulators were now closely watching for long-term risks, and drugs had to prove not only that they worked but also that they protected your heart and overall health. In this section you will see how these medications reflected a major shift toward safer design, clearer oversight, and a stronger focus on understanding how each drug worked inside your body.

>> **Sibutramine (Meridia):** Sibutramine came onto the market in 1997 and worked by changing the levels of three important brain chemicals: serotonin, norepinephrine, and dopamine. As you have learned, these chemicals help control your appetite, mood, and energy. Sibutramine kept these chemicals active longer by blocking their "reuptake," which is the process your brain uses to pull the hormones back in after they are released. When these chemicals

stayed active, you felt less hungry and more satisfied with smaller meals. At first this seemed promising, and many people lost weight on it. But a large study called the SCOUT trial (Sibutramine Cardiovascular OUTcomes trial) found that sibutramine increased the risk of heart attacks and strokes, especially in people who already had heart disease. Because of this danger, the drug was pulled from the market in 2010. This is not a medication you can take today, and you would not want to, because the safety risks were real and serious.

» **Orlistat (Xenical):** Orlistat was approved in 1999 and works in a very different way from earlier weight-loss drugs. Instead of acting on your brain, it works right in your gut by blocking an enzyme called lipase that breaks down fat. When this enzyme is blocked, your body absorbs less fat from the food you eat, and some of that fat passes through your gut, is packaged into your poop, and is evacuated when you use the toilet. This is what is meant by *local action* — the drug does not travel through your bloodstream or affect your heart or nervous system. That lower risk is the reason orlistat is still available today. But because undigested fat has to leave your body, many people experience oily stools, gas, or urgent bathroom trips. You can still get orlistat in prescription strength as Xenical or buy a lower dose over the counter under the name Alli.

» **Exenatide (Byetta):** Byetta arrived in 2005 as a medication for type 2 diabetes, not weight loss. It is part of a group of drugs called GLP-1 receptor agonists (GLP-RAs).

GLP stands for *glucagon-like peptide*. This means it copies a hormone your body already makes to help control blood sugar, appetite, and digestion. This type of drug can also slow the emptying of food contents from your stomach.

When people started using Byetta, doctors noticed that many of them were losing weight without trying. This happened because GLP-1 hormones slow digestion, increase feelings of fullness, and help regulate hunger signals in your brain. That surprise benefit opened the door to a whole new way of thinking about weight-loss medication. It also led to the development of newer GLP-1 medicines like semaglutide and tirzepatide, which are the medications reshaping obesity care today. You can read more about these newer drug developments below and in focus in Chapter 2.

2010s to present day: Mulling over modern options

The 2010s to today have brought some of the biggest breakthroughs we have ever seen in weight-loss medicine. Researchers finally began creating treatments that work with your natural biology instead of fighting against it. The results from this paradigm shift in weight-loss care have been more effective and often much safer than older strategies. In this section you will see how each medication fits into this new era and what you should know before deciding whether one of them is right for you.

>> **Lorcaserin (Belviq):** Belviq was approved in 2012 as a medication to help you feel full sooner and eat less. It worked by gently activating a serotonin receptor in your brain that helps control appetite, and the goal was to create a safer option than older drugs that affected serotonin in riskier ways. At first it looked promising because early studies did not show the heart problems seen with fenfluramine. Over time, however, new safety monitoring raised concerns about a possible link to cancer. Belviq was withdrawn after long-term safety data showed a slightly higher rate of cancer diagnoses in people taking the drug versus those taking a placebo.

WARNING

In a large five-year randomized clinical trial with about 12,000 participants, 7.7 percent of people taking lorcaserin were diagnosed with cancer compared to 7.1 percent in the placebo group. The range of cancers that occurred more often in the lorcaserin group included pancreatic, colorectal, and lung cancer. Because of this safety concern, the manufacturer voluntarily withdrew Belviq from the U.S. market in 2020, and it is no longer available. This is a drug you cannot and should not take now, and it is a good example of why long-term follow-up matters so much when new medications come out.

>> **Naltrexone/bupropion (Contrave):** Contrave was approved in 2014 and is still available today for many patients. It combines two medicines that work together to help you control hunger and reduce cravings. Bupropion increases the activity of dopamine and norepinephrine in your brain, which can help you feel more in control of your eating choices. Naltrexone blocks opioid receptors, which plays a role in reducing the urge to snack for comfort or reward. When these two drugs are paired, they help some people feel less driven by cravings and more able to stick to a plan. Contrave can raise blood pressure and can also affect your mood, so your doctor will monitor you closely to be sure it is safe for you. This is a medication you may be prescribed today, but it requires careful oversight to keep you healthy.

>> **Phentermine/topiramate ER (Qsymia):** Qsymia was approved in 2012 and combines two medications to help you eat less and feel full sooner. Phentermine helps reduce your appetite and gives you a small boost in energy. Topiramate, which is also used to treat migraines, can make certain foods taste less appealing and helps you feel satisfied with smaller portions. Together they create a stronger effect than either medication alone. Qsymia works well for many people, but it can cause birth defects if taken during

pregnancy, which makes it unsafe for anyone who could become pregnant without reliable contraception. If you are a woman of childbearing age, your doctor will require pregnancy testing and consistent birth control before prescribing Qsymia. This medication is still available today, but it must be used with real caution and close follow-up.

>> **GLP-1 and GIP/GLP-1 receptor agonists:** The biggest change in modern weight-loss medicine came with the arrival of injectable GLP-RA drugs, which began with liraglutide in 2014 and grew massively with semaglutide in 2021. Similar in mechanism of action to Byetta (exenatide), these medications copy natural GLP hormones that your gut releases after you eat. They help your brain recognize fullness sooner, reduce hunger between meals, and slow stomach emptying so you stay satisfied longer. They also help keep your blood sugar steady, which can reduce cravings and prevent energy crashes. Tirzepatide, which was approved as Zepbound, goes a step further by activating not only GLP-1 but also another hormone called GIP.

TECHNICAL STUFF

GIP stands for glucose-dependent insulinotropic polypeptide.

It is a natural hormone your body releases from the gut when you eat, especially when you eat carbohydrates or fat. GIP helps your pancreas release insulin at the right time, which keeps your blood sugar steady after meals. It also plays a role in appetite and fat metabolism, which is why newer medications that activate both GIP and GLP-1 can lead to even greater weight loss.

We call this new class of GLP-RAs dual-acting drugs because they work on multiple pathways simultaneously. This combination makes it even easier for many people to lose weight because it targets appetite from more than one angle. These medications do not rely on stimulants or harsh ingredients. They work with your natural biology, which is why they have changed what people expect from weight-loss treatment today and why they remain some of the safest and most effective options your doctor can prescribe. Read Chapter 2 for more information about these types of drugs.

Seeing all of these medications side by side is helpful because the history of weight-loss drugs is full of patterns and repeat lessons. Table 1-1 gives you a quick snapshot of when each major drug arrived, how it worked, and why it stayed or disappeared. It also helps you see how safety standards changed over time and why your doctor is so careful about the medications that are used today. This table offers a historical timeline of major weight-loss drugs and their ultimate outcomes.

TABLE 1-1   Historical Timeline of Major Weight-Loss Drugs

Era	Drug	Mechanism	Outcome
1930s	Thyroid hormone	Increases metabolic rate	Still used for hypothyroidism but not for weight loss without deficiency
1930s	DNP	Uncouples oxidative phosphorylation	Banned for fatal side effects
1940s–1950s	Amphetamines	CNS stimulation, appetite suppression	Controlled due to abuse and addiction potential
1960s–1970s	Rainbow pills	1968	FDA crackdown for safety violations
1970s	Phentermine	Appetite suppression	Still in use short-term
1970s	Fenfluramine	Increases serotonin	Withdrawn for heart valve risk
1990s	Fen-Phen (phentermine/ fenfluramine)	Appetite suppression	Withdraw by FDA
2000s	Meridia (sibutramine)	Reuptake inhibition (5HT, NE, DA)	Withdrawn by FDA for heart disease risk
2000s	Byetta (exenatide)	GLP-1 receptor agonist	Still used for diabetes
2010s	Belviq (lorcaserin)	Serotonin 2C agonist	Withdrawn for cancer risk
2010s	Contrave	Bupropion + naltrexone	Still in use, with specific precautions

Understanding Why You Can Safely Rely on Current Medications

After reading about all the strange, risky, and sometimes terrifying things people once tried to lose weight, you might wonder how you can trust any medication today. You may still see powders, cleanses, or other "fat burners" at big box stores or online. Some of these options promise dramatic results but are not backed up with any scientific evidence. It can feel overwhelming, especially when history has shown us that fast results often come with hidden dangers.

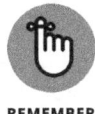

REMEMBER

The good news is that modern weight-loss medications do not follow the old "try it and hope for the best" model. They go through strict review by the FDA, and that process requires years of clinical trials, safety testing, and follow-up after the drug is released. You can find out more about that process in Chapter 2. Chapter 2 specifically outlines the development process of these drugs for you. In Chapter 3 you can explore the importance of using these medications responsibly.

Keep in mind, your doctor is part of your safety net, too. They check your medical history, monitor your labs, watch for side effects, and make sure you are on the right dose or the right medication for your body. This careful oversight is why GLP-RA medications stand on much stronger ground than any creatine blend, energy powder, or "miracle" supplement sold without FDA regulation. You will learn more about how to choose a good doctor who can safely guide you in Chapter 4.

In Chapter 9 we talk about alternatives if medication is not the right path for you. For now, you can feel confident that today's treatments are built on the lessons of the past and designed to protect your health as much as they support your goals.

Examining the Existing Situation

It took a lot of trial and error to reach the medications we have today. This is why understanding the past helps inform your future weight-loss journey. In the next sections you learn why these modern treatments may apply to you, how they work, and how to tell whether they might fit your needs. By the end you will feel more confident, more informed, and better prepared to talk with your doctor about safe and effective options for your own weight-loss journey.

Recognizing the obesity epidemic

Obesity has a specific clinical definition, and it is usually diagnosed when your body mass index, or BMI, reaches 30 or higher. This number is based on your height and weight.

TECHNICAL STUFF

To calculate your BMI, take your weight in pounds, divide it by your height in inches twice, then multiply that number by 703. For example, if you weigh 180 pounds and are 5 feet 4 inches tall (which is 64 inches), your BMI would be $180 \div 64 \div 64 \times 703 = 30.2$, which falls into the obesity range.

REMEMBER

The BMI calculation gives doctors a starting point for understanding your health risks, though it never tells the whole story about you. Obesity does not happen overnight, and it is not something you "catch." Chapter 3: takes you on a deeper dive into this topic. Obesity develops slowly over time, often shaped by biology, environment, stress, and access to care, not by willpower alone. For you, this diagnosis simply means your body is carrying more weight than is healthy for your organs, your joints, and your long-term health. It does not label you as a failure or a problem. It tells your doctor where to begin so you can get the support, tools, and treatment you deserve to improve your health in a safe and sustainable way.

It wasn't until the late 19th and early 20th centuries, when industrialization changed how people lived and worked, that obesity became a widespread concern in developed countries. Food became easier to produce and cheaper to buy, daily movement decreased as jobs became more sedentary, and calorie-dense foods became more available.

By the second half of the 20th century, processed foods, sugary beverages, and fast-food culture spread quickly. Coupled with plummeting rates of physical activity in the 1970s, the obesity rates rose sharply. The proportion of people in the U.S. with obesity has climbed ever since, reaching levels never seen before. Worldwide, obesity rates have more than tripled since 1975, and today more than 1 billion people are living with obesity. In the U.S. alone, over 40 percent of adults meet the clinical definition of obesity, and about 1 in 5 children do as well.

Experts continue to raise the alarm because obesity increases the risk of type 2 diabetes, heart disease, stroke, certain cancers, and early death. If your doctor tells you that you fall into this category, it simply means your health risks are higher than they need to be. For example, people with obesity are about six times more likely to develop type 2 diabetes, and cardiovascular disease is two to three times more common in this group. You are not being judged; you are being given information that can help you take steps to protect your long-term health. And the good news is that even modest weight loss, around 5 to 10 percent of your body weight, can lower these risks in meaningful ways.

Eyeing the global trend in weight-loss management

Weight-loss medications now play a larger role in obesity care than ever before, especially with the rapid rise of GLP-RA medications. Updated medical guidelines recognize GLP-RAs as legitimate, safe treatments alongside lifestyle changes. Part of this global trend in obesity has been severe or morbid obesity. When patients fail lifestyle and medication management or develop severe comorbid conditions (having two or more health conditions or diseases) that cannot be controlled due to excess weight, one of the emerging solutions is bariatric surgery. You can learn more about the indications and options for surgery in Chapter 10.

TIP

These weight-change trends are important because they show a major shift in how the medical community understands obesity. For decades people were told to "eat less and move more," even though many did this and still struggled. The growing use of these medications highlights the reality that obesity is not simply a willpower issue but a chronic, biologically driven condition that often needs medical support. This shift also reflects the fact that traditional methods alone have not kept pace with rising obesity rates around the world. As more people gain access to treatments that actually target the underlying biology, weight-loss medications may finally offer a real chance to turn the tide. For you, this means there are more safe, effective tools available than ever before, and you no longer have to fight this battle on your own.

Zeroing In on your motivations for weight loss

Your motivations are the foundation of your weight-loss journey because they help you understand what you truly want and why you are working toward change. When you connect your goals to something meaningful, it becomes easier to stay focused and to be patient with yourself along the way. Because you know *why* you want to make a change, it becomes easier to stay committed on the hard days and celebrate progress on the good ones. Your motivations also help you set realistic expectations, which you will explore more in Chapter 3, and they can guide the conversations you have with your doctor in Chapter 4. There is no right or wrong reason to want to lose weight. What matters is that your reasons belong to you and support your well-being.

See if you relate to the following reasons people want to lose weight:

» **Improving your health:** This is one of the most common reasons people want to lose weight, and it's valid. Health concerns like high blood pressure, high blood sugar, joint pain, sleep apnea, or increased risk of heart disease can feel scary or overwhelming. Losing even a small amount of weight can lower these risks, reduce inflammation, improve sleep, and help you feel more in control of your health. Your doctor can help you figure out which health issues are most affected by weight so you know exactly what you are working toward.

» **Having more energy:** Feeling tired or sluggish is frustrating, especially when it makes it harder to enjoy your day. Extra weight can strain your joints, increase total body/systemic inflammation, and make your body work harder to move and breathe. As you lose weight, many people notice they sleep better, breathe more easily, and feel more energetic during normal activities. More energy helps you stay active, which also supports long-term weight maintenance.

» **Feeling more confident in your body:** Wanting to feel comfortable and confident in your own skin is a natural motivation. Confidence can influence how you show up at work, in relationships, or even in daily social situations. When weight loss helps you feel more at ease in your body, it can improve self-esteem and help you reconnect with activities or clothes you may have avoided. This is about feeling like yourself again, not meeting anyone else's standard.

>> **Reducing physical discomfort:** Carrying extra weight can put pressure on your knees, hips, back, and feet leading to osteoarthritis. Excess weight can make it harder to climb stairs, walk long distances, or stand for long periods. Even modest weight loss can reduce joint pain, improve mobility, and help you move more freely. This creates a positive cycle where less pain leads to more movement, which supports your health even further.

>> **Being able to participate fully in life:** Maybe you want to travel more comfortably, keep up with your kids or grandkids, or return to past hobbies you used to love. Extra weight can make everyday activities feel harder or less enjoyable. Weight loss can help you regain stamina, flexibility, and confidence in physical activities you want to do. When you can participate more easily, life often feels fuller and more fun.

>> **Preventing future health problems:** Some people are motivated by family history or early signs of conditions like diabetes or heart disease. You might see what loved ones have gone through and want to change your own path. Weight loss can lower your long-term risk for many chronic diseases and may help delay or prevent conditions that seem to run in families. This gives you more control over your future health.

You can how far weight-loss treatments have come and which options are actually safe and available today. The medications you can use now are very different from the risky treatments of the past. These state-of-the-art GLP-RA therapies are supported by real science and strong safety monitoring. In Chapter 2 you can take a closer look at these modern options, how they work, and what they can offer you, so stay tuned.

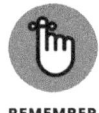

REMEMBER

Different people approach weight loss in different ways, and this book helps you see how each option fits into the bigger picture of your own journey and explore which evidence-based, safe options that are worth your time. When you want to dig deeper into the hows, whys, and why-nots of using medications safely and responsibly, Chapter 3 walks you through exactly what to consider before starting anything. If you are curious about how medications work best when paired with real-life habits, Chapter 5 shows you how nutrition, movement, sleep, and stress management amplify the benefits of treatment. And if you ever find yourself in a spot where medications are not the right choice or do not work for you, Chapter 9 offers practical guidance on supplements, exercise, and eating patterns that can still move you toward your goals.

Chapter **2**

Exploring the Formulations

W eight-loss medications have revolutionized the management of obesity and obesity-related metabolic disorders. They finally address the underlying biology that drives hunger, cravings, and energy balance rather than relying on willpower alone. These medications can help you lose meaningful amounts of weight, improve blood sugar control, lower blood pressure, and reduce long-term health risks in ways that many older treatments simply could not. With the long history of unsafe or ineffective weight-loss remedies, it is understandable to wonder how you can trust the medications available today. The development and approval of these drugs involve a rigorous scientific and regulatory process. In short, the U.S. Food and Drug Administration (FDA) uses an approval process for new drugs designed to ensure safety and effectiveness of each medication for the specific diagnosis it is intending to treat.

TIP

Because there are so many medications out there now, it really helps to understand the difference between drugs approved specifically for weight loss and those approved for type 2 diabetes that happen to cause weight loss as a bonus. One of the biggest breakthroughs in both areas has been a group of medications called GLP-1 receptor agonists, or GLP-RAs. These drugs work with your body's own hormones to help you feel full sooner, steady your blood sugar, and naturally eat less, which is why they've become so popular for both weight loss and diabetes management. These have gained popularity due to their effective weight-loss and metabolic benefits, especially for type 2 diabetes.

In this chapter, you can put any questions about safety to rest by exploring the drug development process for weight-loss medications under the FDA. And you can not only see the science behind these drugs but also gain valuable knowledge about how they actually work, referred to as the *mechanism of action*. I also provide you with practical, real-world tips on tailoring your choice of medicine to your specific and personal needs and answer some questions regarding the safety of brand name medicines versus commonly available compounded options. Finally, you get a sneak peak at the options for future, not-yet-approved weight-loss medicines, which are likely to become available in the next ten years.

Outlining the Medication Development Process

Developing a weight-loss medication involves many stages of research and testing. Most of the work happens long before anything reaches the FDA or you as the patient. Scientists begin with basic laboratory research where they test ideas, study how the body controls appetite and metabolism, and identify compounds that might safely influence those systems. After they find a promising molecule, it goes through years of early testing: first in computer models, then in cells, and finally in animals to see how it behaves in the body. If the results look safe and effective, researchers move on to small human studies to learn how the drug is absorbed, how long it stays in your system, and what side effects might appear. This early phase alone can take many years, sometimes even a decade, before a medication is ready to begin the formal FDA review process. At this point, the drug finally enters the long pipeline of clinical trials required for FDA review. These sections help you understand exactly how this process all works.

Following the FDA approval process

The FDA has a rigorous and lengthy process for drug approval. This step-by-step system is designed to make sure medicines are safe and work well before people can use them. The different phases allow for scientists to check for short- and long-term benefits of the drug, determine the optimal drug dose and frequency of giving yourself the medicine, and verify whether the drug has any potential side effects.

The FDA new drug approval process follows these regimented steps:

1. **Preclinical Testing:** In this first stage, researchers study the drug in the lab and in animals to learn how it behaves in the body. They look at how the drug is absorbed, how it is broken down, and whether it shows any early signs of toxicity. This step helps scientists decide if the drug is safe enough to even consider testing in humans.

2. **Phase 1 Clinical Trials:** The drug is tested on a small group of healthy volunteers (20 to 100). The goal here is to understand basic safety, find the right dose range, and identify any early side effects. This phase indicates whether humans can safely take this medication at all.

3. **Phase 2 Clinical Trials:** After basic safety is established, the drug is given to a larger group of people (100 to 300) who has the condition. Researchers begin to evaluate whether the drug works as intended and continue to monitor for safety concerns. This phase helps determine which doses are most effective and whether the benefits seem promising enough to move forward.

4. **Phase 3 Clinical Trials:** The drug is tested on an even larger group (1,000 to 3,000-plus). Researchers compare the drug to existing treatments or to a placebo to confirm that it truly works. They also track a wider range of side effects and learn how the drug performs in people with different ages, backgrounds, and medical histories. This strategy helps to describe the drug's effectiveness, monitor side effects, and compare it to commonly used treatments.

5. **FDA Review:** When all trial phases are complete, the company submits a New Drug Application (NDA) to the FDA with thousands of pages of data. FDA experts review the evidence to decide whether the medication is safe, effective, and properly manufactured. This is the point where the FDA can approve the drug, request more research, or deny approval.

6. **Phase 4 (Post-Marketing Surveillance):** Even after a drug is approved, the monitoring does not stop. The medication is tracked in the general population to see how it performs in real-world use, including rare side effects that may not appear in clinical trials. This ongoing review helps ensure long-term safety and can lead to label updates or, in rare cases, withdrawal from the market.

Working through FDA evaluation metrics

The FDA evaluates new weight–loss drugs based on several key metrics to decide if they should be approved for the market:

>> **Efficacy (weight-loss percentage):** The drug should show a clinically meaningful amount of weight loss. For the weight loss to be meaningful, the

FDA typically reviews whether those who took the medication showed at least a 5 percent greater reduction in body weight after one year compared to those who took the placebo.

>> **Safety profile:** The medication must demonstrate an acceptable safety profile, with no serious or unacceptable side effects outweighing the benefits. The medication must show that its benefits outweigh its risks, and that any side effects are manageable and predictable. In weight-loss trials, the FDA looks for side effects such as heart valve damage, which happened with fenfluramine, or dangerous increases in heart rate and blood pressure, which were seen with some stimulant medications. They also watch for psychiatric symptoms like severe mood changes or suicidal thoughts, which have shown up in rare cases with bupropion-containing drugs. Serious gastrointestinal problems, such as pancreatitis or severe nausea and vomiting, have also raised red flags in past studies of metabolic medications. If a drug shows patterns of organ damage, cardiac strain, cancer signals, or life-threatening reactions, the FDA will not approve it or may remove it from the market later. These safeguards are in place so you never receive a medication with risks that are hidden or ignored.

>> **Sustained results:** The weight-loss effect should be maintained with medication use over a long period, usually confirmed by at least 12 months of data.

>> **Improvement in related health markers:** Benefits like improved blood pressure, blood sugar control, or cholesterol levels may strengthen the case for approval.

>> **Risk-benefit analysis:** The FDA weighs the overall benefits of weight loss and improved health against potential risks or adverse events to ensure the medication is safe for widespread use.

HEALTH MARKERS: DRAWING A PICTURE OF YOUR PHYSICAL WELL-BEING

Your health markers are like a snapshot of what is happening inside your body, helping you see things you cannot always feel, such as blood sugar levels, cholesterol, inflammation, and organ function. Tracking these numbers gives you and your doctor a clearer picture of how weight-loss efforts are affecting your overall health, not just the number on the scale. To learn how to monitor these markers and use them to maintain long-term success, you can read more in Chapter 6.

Understanding what "sustained results" means for your weight loss

Most studies for weight-loss drugs which show "sustained" results mean that you must continue the medication indefinitely. If you stop your weight-loss medicine, most studies indicate that you will regain at least a percentage of the weight you had previously lost.

The latest evidence suggests that most people who stop GLP receptor agonist medications will regain weight approximately eight to twenty weeks later. Average weight regain among participants in one meta-analysis study was:

>> **3.3 pounds** (1.5 kg) at 8 weeks

>> **3.9 pounds** (1.76 kg) at 12 weeks

>> **5.5 pounds** (2.5 kg) at 20 weeks

>> **5.1 pounds** (2.3 kg) at 26 weeks

>> **5.45 pounds** (2.47 kg) at 52 weeks

Despite this gradual regain, individuals who had previously used weight-loss medications still maintained a net weight loss compared to their pre-treatment baseline at the fifty-two-week mark. Thus, even if you stop your weight-loss medication, there is a chance you may experience sustained benefit. The likelihood of sustaining weight loss after discontinuing weight-loss medications is enhanced by commitment to appropriate lifestyle choices. (See Chapter 5 for more info on making lifestyle changes.)

TIP

Some companies that design medications for weight loss or for type 2 diabetes do not always build in the diet and lifestyle support you actually need to succeed with these treatments. This means you might receive a prescription without the guidance that helps the medication work its best, even though most weight-loss medications are far more effective when paired with changes in eating habits, movement, sleep, and stress. Some medications will not reach their full potential unless you make those adjustments, and others may cause challenges that are easier to manage when you have a solid lifestyle plan in place. That is why learning how to integrate these changes into your journey is so important and why staying curious about what your body needs will help you sustain better results. (See Chapter 8 to better understand how to navigate medicine challenges you may experience by implementing new lifestyle management strategies.)

Exploring the Science behind Weight-Loss Medications

Understanding how medications work can help you better understand which ones might best meet your needs. These sections arm you with information so you can have a productive discussion with your doctor about taking these medications.

How GLP-1 meds work

Glucagon-like peptide-1 (GLP-1) medications have transformed obesity treatment by leveraging the body's natural hormonal pathways to control appetite and blood sugar. GLP-1 is an incretin hormone released after eating, which stimulates insulin secretion, slows stomach (gastric) emptying (pushing food from your stomach into the intestine for digestion), and reduces hunger signals in the brain. Researchers synthesized GLP-1 receptor agonists that mimic this hormone but last longer in the body, thereby promoting weight loss and improving blood sugar control in people with type 2 diabetes. These medications not only reduce caloric intake by increasing satiety but also improve metabolic health by lowering blood glucose levels and improving insulin sensitivity.

REMEMBER

GLP-1 medications like liraglutide and semaglutide work by copying a natural gut hormone that helps you feel full sooner, slows down how quickly your stomach empties, and steadies your blood sugar so you are not constantly battling hunger. When a medication, like tirzepatide, activates both GLP-1 and another hormone, GIP (glucose-dependent insulinotropic polypeptide), it adds another hormone that boosts your body's ability to regulate appetite and use energy more efficiently. Together these actions help you eat less without feeling deprived, and they make it easier for your body to shift toward weight loss. Any medication that uses GLP-1 alone or GLP-1 plus GIP is considered a GLP receptor agonist, or GLP-RA, which simply means it activates the same receptors your natural gut hormones use.

GLP receptor agonists bind to receptors in the pancreas and brain, triggering a cascade of responses that regulate hunger and metabolism. These responses help you achieve weight loss because they are designed to

>> **Decrease appetite and provide you with the feeling of fullness:** The medications do this, in part, by slowing the emptying of the stomach. So, theoretically, you decrease your total daily calories consumed by promoting the feeling of fullness throughout the day.

>> **Control blood sugar:** Insulin is a hormone your body makes to move sugar (glucose) out of the bloodstream and into your cells, where it's used for energy. These GLP-RA medications help your body release insulin at the right time, such as when you eat, so blood sugar rises are handled more efficiently. The GLP-RA medicines also reduce glucagon, a hormone that signals the liver to release extra sugar when it isn't needed. By keeping blood sugar levels steadier, these medications help prevent energy crashes and strong hunger cues, which can make weight loss feel more manageable over time.

Together, these effects create a powerful tool for managing obesity and diabetes. However, these medications do have possible side effects. You can learn more about side effects and managing them in Chapter 8.

WARNING

GLP receptor agonist medications are not recommended for people who have a personal or family history of a rare thyroid cancer called medullary thyroid carcinoma, or a genetic condition known as multiple endocrine neoplasia type 2. These conditions are uncommon, but they matter because this class of medications has been linked to thyroid tumors in animal studies. Your healthcare provider will review your personal and family medical history to be sure these medications are a safe option for you.

TIP

Most commonly, you will be prescribed a GLP–RA in the injectable formulation. This delivery system allows for slow, steady release of the drug, providing prolonged benefits with weekly or daily dosing compared to taking oral formulations of the drug.

SPECIAL DELIVERY: WHY INJECTIONS WORK BEST

Injected weight-loss medications work better than pills because they bypass the digestive system and go directly into the bloodstream, allowing the medication to be absorbed fully and consistently. This steady delivery makes it easier to accurately copy natural gut hormones like GLP-1 and GIP, which are quickly broken down if taken by mouth. As a result, injections provide more reliable appetite control, longer-lasting effects, and more consistent weight loss compared with oral versions.

How combination GLP-1 and GIP meds work

GLP-1 works by attaching to GLP-1 receptors in the brain, stomach, and pancreas. When these receptors are activated, your brain receives stronger "I'm full" signals, your stomach empties more slowly, and your pancreas releases insulin in a more controlled way, all of which reduce hunger and help prevent overeating.

GIP works by attaching to GIP receptors found in the brain, pancreas, and fat tissue. Activation of these receptors improves how your body responds to insulin, helps regulate how calories are stored versus burned, and appears to further quiet appetite signals in the brain. When GIP and GLP-1 receptors are activated together, they reinforce each other's effects, leading to better appetite control, fewer cravings, and more efficient use of energy that supports sustained weight loss.

How other weight-loss meds work

These earlier weight-loss medications primarily work by suppressing appetite or reducing calorie absorption, but they generally produce less weight loss compared with newer GLP-based therapies. While still helpful for some patients, the following medications highlight how much obesity treatment has evolved toward safer, more effective long-term options:

>> **Orlistat:** Approved in 1999 for weight loss and weight maintenance, it works in the gut by blocking the absorption of some dietary fat so fewer calories are taken in. People lose about 3 to 5 percent of their body weight. Because the fat passes through your digestive system instead, side effects often include oily stools, gas, or urgent bowel movements, especially after high-fat meals.

>> **Phentermine–topiramate:** This combination works mainly by reducing your appetite and helping you feel full sooner. Many people lose around 8 to 10 percent of their body weight and sometimes more at higher doses. Side effects can include a racing heart, dry mouth, tingling in the hands or feet, trouble sleeping, or changes in mood or concentration. You should avoid this medication if you have glaucoma, overactive thyroid disease, or have recently taken certain antidepressants.

>> **Naltrexone–bupropion:** Approved in 2014 for chronic weight management, this medication targets hunger and cravings in the brain, which can be especially helpful if emotional or reward-driven eating is a struggle for you. Average weight loss is about 5 to 9 percent of body weight. Common side effects include nausea, headache, dry mouth, and sometimes increased anxiety or blood pressure. It is not a good option if you have a seizure disorder, uncontrolled high blood pressure, an eating disorder, or regularly use opioid medications.

>> **Phentermine (alone):** This drug works by stimulating your nervous system to suppress appetite and is approved only for short-term use since 1959. People often lose about 3 to 5 percent of body weight over a few months. Side effects can include jitteriness, insomnia, increased heart rate, and feeling "amped up." Because of these effects, it is not meant for long-term use and should be avoided if you have heart disease, glaucoma, or thyroid problems.

Detailing the Weight-Loss Medications Available

The United States has approved several GLP-1 receptor agonists for weight loss and type 2 diabetes. Some medications, like semaglutide, are used for both conditions and go by different brand names: Ozempic for diabetes and Wegovy for weight loss. You've probably heard of these brands because semaglutide is among the most widely prescribed and studied, showing significant weight reduction in clinical trials. However, you can find a range of medications to choose from, each drug varying in dosing frequency, efficacy, and side-effect profile, providing you with options tailored to your specific needs. We break down these medications in the following sections, dividing them by condition so you can zero in on the best fit for you.

TIP

When looking at your options, consider whether you can incorporate a daily medicine to your routine or if a weekly injection might be easier for you to remember.

Breaking down medications approved in the U.S. for weight loss

Currently, the FDA has approved several medications specifically for weight loss. Although Wegovy (semaglutide) and Saxenda (liraglutide) are the most prominent GLP-1 receptor agonists used for obesity management, other medications beyond GLPs, like orlistat (which blocks fat absorption) and phentermine-topiramate (a combination that suppresses appetite), also hold FDA approval for weight loss.

All weight-loss medications offer varying mechanisms of action (ways they work with your body) and degrees of efficacy (how well they work). So which one your doctor may prescribe depends on your individual patient profile and health conditions. To make comparing these drugs easier, you can look at Table 2-1 to see which drugs best fit your situation so you can make an informed decision with your doctor.

TABLE 2-1 FDA-Approved Meds for Weight Loss

Generic (brand)	Mechanism	Administration	Percent weight loss	Sustainability
Semaglutide (Wegovy)	GLP-1	Weekly injectable	15%	
Liraglutide (Saxenda)	GLP-1	Daily injectable	8%	
Tirzepatide (Zepbound)	GLP-1 and GIP	Daily injectable	20%	
Exenatide (Byetta)	GLP-1	Twice-daily injectable	5 to 10%	
Orlistat (Alli [OTC], Xenical)	Reduces fat absorption	Oral	5 to 7%	
Phentermine-topiramate (Qsymia)	Appetite uppressant	Oral	9 to 10%	
Naltrexone-bupropion (Contrave)	Acts on appetite regulation centers	Oral	5 to 8%	

Looking at medications approved in the U.S. for type 2 diabetes

GLP-1 receptor agonists were originally pioneered and received FDA approval to treat type 2 diabetes. Medications like Ozempic (semaglutide), Victoza (liraglutide), and Trulicity (dulaglutide) help lower blood sugar with the added benefit of promoting weight loss. These drugs have become part of standard diabetes care because they reduce cardiovascular risks and improve glucose control. You can compare these medications in Table 2-2 and discuss them with your doctor. (Chapter 4 focuses on seeking healthcare guidance and best tips to adhere to your provider dosing schedule.)

Because many of these medications have demonstrated robust weight-loss properties, some have received separate FDA approvals to be used specifically for obesity treatment, which we cover in the earlier section, "Breaking down medications approved in the U.S. for weight loss." You can review these medications in greater detail using Table 2-2, below.

TECHNICAL STUFF

Studies have been published regarding high-dose strategies using GLP-1s. The STEP-UP Phase 3b trial recently tested once-weekly high-dose semaglutide (7.2 mg), which produced 18.7 percent average weight loss compared with 15.6 percent at a dose of 2.4 mg and 3.9 percent with placebo. Odds of achieving at least 25 percent weight loss were more than twofold higher with the escalated dose.

TABLE 2-2 **FDA-Approved Meds for Type 2 Diabetes**

Generic (brand)	Mechanism	Administration	Percent weight loss	Sustainability
Semaglutide (Ozempic)	GLP-1	Weekly injectable	15%	
Semaglutide (Rybelsus)	GLP-1	Daily oral	5 to 10%	
Liraglutide (Victoza)	GLP-1	Daily injectable	8%	
Tirzepatide (Mounjaro)	GLP-1 and GIP	Daily injectable	20%	
Exenatide (Bydureon)	GLP-1	Once-weekly injectable	5 to 10%	
Dulaglutide (Trulicity)	GLP-1	Weekly injectable	2 to 6%	

Comparing Brand Name Medications and Compound Options

The popularity of GLP-1 medications has been unparalleled when compared to other medications in the U.S. This has, in turn, led to drug shortages from several manufacturers. These brand-name drug shortages have sparked interest amongst many people in the use of non-FDA approved, compounded formulations of semaglutide and other GLP RAs.

Compounding pharmacies create customized medication doses or combinations not commercially available, often at lower cost. However, these compounded drugs differ chemically from FDA-approved versions, sometimes lacking the same stabilizers or purity standards. If you're considering compounded options, use these sections to understand how these options could vary in efficacy and safety compared to branded drugs.

Getting an opinion from the FDA

We get it. You may not care much for "big brother" telling you what you can and can't do, but the FDA is tasked with keeping you safe. And while Aunt Martha may tell you how great she's doing after trying out the newest compound formulation, one anecdote can't outweigh the rigorous testing and scrutiny the FDA puts into new medications.

WARNING

The FDA has issued warnings about compounded versions of semaglutide and other GLP-1 receptor agonists because these products do not go through the same safety and quality checks as FDA-approved medications. Contamination does not necessarily mean "dirty," but it can include problems such as bacteria or mold introduced during preparation, particles from improper mixing, or chemical impurities if ingredients are not handled or stored correctly. For patients, this can translate into infections at injection sites, unexpected side effects, or inconsistent dosing that affects how well the medication works.

The FDA also cautions against compounding these medications when there is no medical necessity, such as when an FDA-approved version is readily available. Compounding is intended for specific situations, like when a patient cannot tolerate an ingredient in the approved drug or needs a different dose or formulation. Using compounded versions outside of these situations may fall outside of regulatory standards, which is why patients are encouraged to discuss risks, benefits, and alternatives carefully with their healthcare provider.

TIP

You can read more about the FDA's concerns with these medications at https://www.fda.gov/drugs/postmarket-drug-safety-information-patients-and-providers/fdas-concerns-unapproved-glp-1-drugs-used-weight-loss. And you can review the FDA's BeSafeRx campaign for resources to safely buy prescription medicines online at https://www.fda.gov/drugs/buying-using-medicine-safely/besaferx-your-source-online-pharmacy-information. These resources can help you determine the risks of compounded forms of weight-loss medicines as alternatives to the FDA-approved formulations.

THE COMPOUND CONUNDRUM

People often turn to compounded medications when FDA-approved options are too expensive, hard to find, or temporarily unavailable. During periods of high demand, some pharmacies were able to offer compounded versions that felt like a more accessible alternative, especially for patients eager to start treatment rather than wait. Cost differences and supply shortages are usually the biggest drivers, not necessarily a belief that compounds work better.

That said, compounded medications are not the same as FDA-approved injectables. They may use different formulations, doses, or salt forms, and they are not required to go through the same testing for safety, effectiveness, or how long the drug stays active in the body. Because of this, results can be less predictable, side effects may differ, and the medication's half-life and consistency may not match what was studied in clinical trials. For these reasons, it is important for patients to approach any compounded medication thoughtfully and to have a clear conversation with a knowledgeable healthcare provider about risks, benefits, and alternatives.

Noting the chemical difference

FDA-approved GLP-1 drugs undergo extensive testing to optimize their chemical stability, absorption, and shelf life. In contrast, compounded versions may use different inactive ingredients or preparation methods, which can change how the medication behaves once it is in the body. For example, if a compounded formulation is absorbed too quickly, a person might feel strong nausea or appetite suppression for a day or two, followed by several days where the medication seems to wear off early. This uneven exposure can make weight loss less consistent. Proper formulation matters because it helps ensure both safety and reliable results.

Looking at related risks

FDA-approved medications carry known safety profiles based on large clinical trials. Compounded drugs, however, often lack such comprehensive data. Risks include dosing inaccuracies, contamination (with bacteria), and inconsistent drug effects on your body. Patients using compounded versions may face unforeseen adverse effects or reduced therapeutic benefits. Your doctor should weigh these risks with you when considering compounding as an option.

According to the FDA's Adverse Event Reporting System (FAERS), compounded GLP-1 receptor agonists exhibit 2.8 times greater odds for developing side effects like abdominal pain when compared to brand-name, FDA-approved (non-compounded) drug formulations. A recent pharmacovigilance study analyzed FDA adverse-event reports for compounded GLP-1 products and found substantially higher safety risks compared with FDA-approved formulations. Compounded versions were linked to increased rates of abdominal pain, diarrhea, gallbladder disease, and even suicidality. Product quality issues were also prominent, including manufacturing errors and preparation problems, with risk ratios higher than brand-name, FDA-approved drugs. Hospitalization odds were more than twice as high among users of compounded GLP-1s.

REMEMBER

You should know that adverse event reporting is likely incomplete and underestimated because compounders are not legally required to submit data to the FDA. These findings raise concerns about the safety and consistency of unregulated compounded products. Bottom line: compounded GLP-1s carry higher and underreported risks that you must recognize. These findings parallel FAERS data which suggests that you will be at increased risk for cholecystitis (gallbladder inflammation), suicidality, or hospitalization. Table 2-3 summarizes some of the key differences between the FDA-approved and the compounded weight-loss medicine options.

TIP

When evaluating a compounding pharmacy verify the following key credentials to ensure that your medicine meets minimum safety and quality standards.

» Confirm that the compounding pharmacy possesses a Pharmacy Compounding Accreditation Board (PCAB) certificate, which is widely recognized as the gold standard for signaling adherence to rigorous quality and safety standards.

» The pharmacy should also comply with USP guidelines, including:

- USP <795> for nonsterile compounding,
- USP <797> for sterile compounding, and
- USP <800> for hazardous drug handling, particularly under 503A licensing.

» The compounding pharmacy must also adhere to the Drug Quality and Security Act (DQSA), which governs the distinction between patient-specific compounding (503A) and outsourcing facilities (503B).

» If compounding GLP-1 medications during non-shortage periods, the compounding pharmacy must use FDA-registered bulk drug substances and have appropriate FDA approvals or registration.

» High-quality compounders should provide Certificates of Analysis (COAs) for their formulations, confirming identity, potency, and purity — ideally using USP-standard methods such as HPLC, pH testing, and clarity assessments.

TABLE 2-3   **Comparing Brand Names and Compounds**

Category	FDA-Approved Semaglutide (Wegovy/Ozempic)	Compounded Semaglutide
Formulation	Semaglutide (base)	Often semaglutide sodium or acetate (research-grade)
FDA Approval	Yes	No
Clinical Trial Data	Extensive Phase III trials	No large, peer-reviewed clinical trials
Average Weight Loss	About 15% or more over 68 weeks (Wegovy)	Unknown; not validated in controlled trials
Manufacturing Standards	Strict FDA oversight; Good Manufacturing Practices (GMP)	Varies by pharmacy; not held to same FDA standards
Dosing Consistency	Precise and standardized dosing	Potential for dosing variability
Safety Profile	Well-documented side-effect data	Unknown or variable safety profile
Known Side Effects	Nausea, vomiting, diarrhea, constipation, gallbladder issues	Similar risks possible; additional risks due to impurities/dosing

EXPLORING FUTURE ALTERNATIVES TO GLP MEDICATIONS

While GLP-1 receptor agonists are likely to be effective for you, researchers continue exploring novel treatments for obesity. One promising alternative is APHD-012, a small bead that releases sugar in the later part of the small intestine designed to mimic the body's natural satiety signals by targeting the gut-brain connection.

When you ingest this medication on an empty stomach, there is high dose dextrose release. The beads release dextrose, a simple sugar, which is readily absorbed by the intestinal lining. The drug is specifically designed so that this absorption occurs lower in the smaller intestine in an area called the jejunum. This mechanism capitalizes on maximum absorption where glucose transporters are most active. This targeted release can cause a short-term increase in your blood glucose levels compared to other forms of glucose administration. The hope is that by increasing glucose absorption on an empty stomach, you could experience increased levels of insulin secretion for the meal to come.

In addition, there is a theory that this rapid increase in blood glucose may decrease your appetite even before the meal is consumed. This could occur because your intestine absorbed the dextrose carbohydrate leading to your sense of fullness without a high-caloric load from fats, proteins, or other carbohydrates. This approach could provide you with an oral, non-hormonal option to regulate appetite and improve metabolic health without some GLP-associated side effects. Early trials indicate potential, marking an exciting future direction in weight-loss therapeutics.

Practicing Diligence When Choosing Medication

Choosing the right weight–loss medication involves more than just filling a prescription. You must balance efficacy, safety, convenience, and cost, and these tips can help:

>> **Talk to your doctor extensively about your situation.** You and your medical provider must consider your medical history, your other medical conditions, and your current lifestyle when selecting treatment (see Chapter 5 for more about integrating lifestyle changes to your medication regimen). You must also answer two important questions when selecting a weight-loss medication:

- Are you comfortable with receiving an injection method or would you prefer an oral medicine option?

- Will it be easier for you to remember to take a medicine once a day or once a week?

>> **Be prepared to monitor for side effects.** Be prepared to watch for side effects and address them early. Following the medication schedule and lifestyle recommendations closely helps reduce side effects and improves your chances of staying on treatment long enough to see results. For example, increasing the dose too quickly can raise the risk of nausea, vomiting, or fatigue, while allowing your body time to adjust can make the medication much easier to tolerate (see Chapter 8 for tips on recognizing and managing common side effects).

>> **Consider joining Obesity Action Coalition (OAC).** This group can help you stay informed and up-to-date on medical weight-loss solutions (https://www.obesityaction.org/about/purpose/who-we-are/). OAC is a patient-focused education, advocacy, and news on obesity treatment which provides regular updates on FDA-approved medications.

See Chapter 4 for more in-depth details on dosing.

Taking a Look at the Future of Weight-Loss Medications

The future of weight-loss medications looks promising. Researchers are working to improve drug delivery systems, reduce side effects, and enhance efficacy. Trials are underway for triple agonists that activate GLP-1 (a hormone that increases fullness and slows stomach emptying), GIP (a hormone that improves appetite control and how the body uses energy), and glucagon (a hormone that increases calorie burning and energy use) receptors at the same time, with impressive weight-loss results.

At the same time, researchers are studying new weight-loss treatments that work by targeting specific receptors in the gut and brain that help control hunger, fullness, and how the body uses energy. Examples include medications that act on melanocortin receptors in the brain, which play a key role in appetite and energy balance, and opioid and dopamine-related receptors, which are involved in food cravings and reward-driven eating.

In the gut, scientists are exploring receptors linked to bile acids, nutrient sensing, and hormones like peptide YY (PYY) and amylin, which help signal fullness and slow digestion. By targeting these receptors directly, future medications may help regulate appetite and metabolism in new ways, offering alternatives for people who cannot tolerate or do not respond to current GLP–based treatments. Some of these cutting–edge weight–loss medications may become FDA–approved options in the next ten years.

Promising drugs being studied right now include:

» **Cagrilintide plus semaglutide:** A weekly injection studied for obesity and type 2 diabetes, this combination activates GLP-1 receptors to reduce appetite and slow digestion, while also activating amylin pathways that increase fullness and reduce food intake. People in studies lost about 20.4 percent of their total body weight, which puts this therapy close to surgical-level results and makes it one of the most exciting options in late-stage trials.

» **Retatrutide:** A weekly injection being studied for obesity and cardiometabolic disease, it activates three receptors, GLP-1 to reduce appetite, GIP to improve energy use, and glucagon to increase calorie burning. Participants have lost up to 24.2 percent of body weight, making this one of the most powerful medications ever studied for weight loss.

» **Orforglipron:** A daily oral pill studied for obesity and type 2 diabetes, it is a non-peptide GLP-1 receptor agonist, meaning it mimics GLP-1's appetite-reducing effects without requiring an injection. While average weight loss is lower than injectables, many participants achieved 10 to 20 percent weight loss, making this a very promising option for people who strongly prefer pills over shots.

» **Aleniglipron:** A daily oral pill studied for obesity and diabetes, like orforglip-ron, it activates GLP-1 receptors to reduce hunger and improve blood sugar control. Early animal studies show encouraging results, and researchers are hopeful it could expand effective oral treatment options in the future.

» **Mazdutide:** A weekly injection studied for obesity and PCOS, it activates both GLP-1 and glucagon receptors, helping reduce appetite while increas-ing energy use. In studies, people lost about 15.4 percent of body weight, and it performed well compared with semaglutide, making it especially interesting for patients with metabolic or hormonal conditions.

» **Maridebart cafraglutide:** A monthly injection studied for obesity and type 2 diabetes, it stimulates GLP-1 receptors while blocking GIP receptors, a strategy thought to enhance fat loss while maintaining appetite control. Early results show up to 20 percent weight loss, with the added benefit of less frequent dosing.

» **Oral semaglutide:** A daily oral pill studied for overweight and obesity, it uses the same GLP-1 mechanism as injectable semaglutide, reducing appetite and slowing digestion but in pill form. Trials show 13 to 17 percent weight loss, making it one of the most effective oral options studied so far.

» **Survodutide:** A weekly injection studied for obesity, it activates both GLP-1 and glucagon receptors, combining appetite suppression with increased energy expenditure. Participants lost up to 19 percent of body weight, placing it among the stronger next-generation injectables.

» **UBT251:** A weekly injection studied for obesity, this triple agonist activates GLP-1, GIP, and glucagon receptors to reduce hunger, improve metabolism, and increase calorie burning. Early studies show around 15 percent weight loss, and researchers are optimistic as trials continue.

» **Distal jejunal-release dextrose:** A daily oral therapy studied for obesity, rather than acting on hormones directly, it delivers small amounts of sugar to a specific part of the intestine to trigger natural fullness signals and improve metabolic responses. This gut-targeted approach is exciting because it avoids injections and hormones altogether.

» **Bivamelagon:** A daily oral pill studied for hypothalamic obesity, it activates the MC4 receptor in the brain, a key pathway involved in appetite and energy balance. While weight-loss data are still pending, this drug is especially promising for people whose obesity is driven by brain-based signaling disorders.

» **Bimagrumab plus GLP-1 combo:** An injectable combination studied for obesity, this therapy pairs a GLP-1 agonist for appetite control with a drug that helps preserve or increase muscle mass. The goal is not just weight loss, but healthier body composition, which could be a major advancement if results continue to be positive.

These emerging medications show that the future of weight-loss treatment is moving toward more effective, more personalized options. Some future drugs may offer results similar to surgery, while others focus on convenience, such as monthly injections or daily pills. There is likely to be a large number of options and alternatives if you cannot tolerate current GLP-based therapies. Although these treatments are still being studied and are not yet available, they signal that weight-loss care is becoming more targeted, more flexible, and more focused on long-term health rather than quick fixes. Here are the two biggest take-aways:

» **Future injectables may offer the most powerful non-surgical weight loss options available.** New injectable GLP-based medications such as retatrutide have produced weight loss of about 24 percent of total body weight, which is even greater than what we see with tirzepatide. Since tirzepatide already leads to substantial weight loss for many people, this tells us that newer medications may push results even further.

>> **Improved oral medications could give patients meaningful weight loss without the need for injections.** High-dose oral GLP-1 medications, including orforglipron (about 10 15 percent weight loss) and a newer oral form of semaglutide (about 17 percent weight loss), show better results than the currently approved oral GLP-1 medication, Rybelsus. This means pills may soon approach the effectiveness of injections for some people.

WARNING

As of April 2025, the pharmaceutical company Pfizer halted development of danuglipron (PF-06882961), an oral glucagon-like peptide-1 (GLP-1) receptor agonist, which was being investigated for chronic weight management. Danuglipron had successfully progressed through 2 FDA trials (NCT06567327 and NCT06568731) and moved on to Phase 3 trial. During this investigation, a participant was found to develop danuglipron-induced liver injury. Pfizer then discontinued further danuglipron development in the interest of patient safety.

These alternative therapies are also being studied to expand weight-loss options beyond current GLP-based medications:

>> **Gut hormone modulators** aim to enhance the body's natural fullness signals after eating, helping people feel satisfied with less food.

>> **Microbiome-based therapies** focus on changing the balance of gut bacteria to improve metabolism, reduce inflammation, and influence appetite regulation.

>> **Metabolic enzyme inhibitors** work by altering how the body processes or absorbs calories, which can reduce energy storage.

>> Early research into compounds like **APHD-012**, an oral gut-targeted therapy, is especially promising because it may help trigger fullness signals without injections, offering a potential non-hormonal alternative for weight loss.

IN THIS CHAPTER

» **Seeking healthcare provider guidance for follow up and testing**

» **Determining whether you're a candidate for GLP-RA medication**

» **Understanding the risks of weight-loss medicines**

» **Detailing tests you need**

» **Searching for meds on various platforms**

Chapter **3**

Getting Started with GLP-RA Medications

GLP-1 agonist medications have changed the game when it comes to treating obesity and related conditions like type 2 diabetes. If you're considering one of these medications, it's important for you to understand not just the benefits but also how to use them safely, under the right conditions, and with the right support. In this chapter, you will walk through how to recognize if a GLP-1 medication is right for you. You will gain valuable insight and technical know-how to prepare yourself for your weight-loss journey with validated screening tools, the right labs, and what to watch out for along the way.

When you start a GLP-RA medication under the right conditions, you set yourself up for long-term success. Think of this chapter not just as information but as a conversation. We equip you with the info you need so you're empowered to ask questions, advocate for yourself, and make choices with informed confidence.

Soliciting Advice from the Experts

Obesity is a complex, chronic disease. Your weight loss journey is not a simple matter of willpower. That's why expert guidance matters. A Diplomate of the American Board of Obesity Medicine (DABOM) is specially trained to help patients understand whether GLP-1 therapy is appropriate and how to safely manage weight. Making your weight-loss journey a success will take a team!

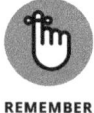

REMEMBER

Studies consistently show that specialized, multidisciplinary approaches to obesity, including the participation of behavioral counselors. Guided medical oversight leads to better weight-loss outcomes and improved metabolic health than standard primary care interventions.

So who should be on your team? We cover the details of each of the following teammates in Chapter 4:

>> A **prescribing clinician,** such as a primary care provider, endocrinologist, gastroenterologist, or obesity medicine specialist

>> A **registered** dietitian to support nutritional goals

>> A **behavioral health provider** to address emotional factors

>> An **exercise professional** to help maintain lean mass and mobility

Before your first injection or pill, ensure your care team:

>> Reviews your full medical and medication history

>> Conducts a thorough physical exam

>> Orders labs for metabolic health and nutritional deficiencies (see the later section, "Getting Appropriate Tests and Screening" for more on what test you might need)

>> Discusses goals, risks, and treatment duration (see the later section, "Understanding the Risks" to check out risks and nutritional deficiencies worth discussing with your team)

>> Explains insurance requirements and coverage options (see Chapter 4 to learn more about navigating health insurance coverage for obesity)

Determining the Need for Weight-Loss Medication

If you're wanting to start weight-loss medications, the first thing you want to know is whether you're a candidate for them. Although you must make this determination with your doctor and every situation is unique, we can outline the qualifying markers your doctor will be looking for. The sections below outline the key factors your doctor will assess when deciding whether weight-loss medication is medically appropriate for you.

REMEMBER

Your need isn't determined solely based on your weight; it's also about your overall health. In general, GLP-RAs, such as semaglutide, are prescribed if your BMI (body mass index) is 30 or more or if your BMI is 27 or more and you have at least one weight-related health condition. Common weight-related health conditions that may qualify you for GLP receptor agonist medications when your BMI is 27 or higher include:

>> Type 2 diabetes or prediabetes

>> High blood pressure (hypertension)

>> High cholesterol or triglycerides (dyslipidemia)

>> Obstructive sleep apnea

>> Heart disease or a history of cardiovascular disease

>> Nonalcoholic fatty liver disease (NAFLD/NASH)

>> Polycystic ovary syndrome (PCOS)

>> Osteoarthritis or chronic joint pain worsened by weight

To get you prepared for what's ahead, we walk you through exactly what to expect when talking to your doctor about your need for GLP-RA medications.

Assessing your BMI

One of the first things your healthcare provider will look at is your body mass index (BMI). The measurement index is not perfect, but it gives you a rough estimate of your body fat based on your height and weight.

To determine your BMI, your doctor will use your height and weight to calculate a simple number that helps guide medical decisions. In most visits, a nurse or medical assistant will measure your height and weight when you check in, often just like at any routine appointment, and your doctor will review the number with you later in a private, nonjudgmental conversation. You do not need a full physical exam just to calculate BMI, and this part of the visit is usually quick and straightforward. Many clinicians are very aware that weight can be a sensitive topic and will focus on health, not appearance.

REMEMBER

BMI helps doctors decide whether weight-loss medications may be medically appropriate, not as a measure of your worth or effort. Certain medications are studied and approved for people above specific BMI thresholds because research shows they are most likely to benefit safely in those groups. The table below shows how BMI ranges relate to medication eligibility, which can help you better understand why your doctor may or may not recommend medication as part of your care.

Table 3-1 shows how your BMI relates to your need for FDA-approved GLP-1 medications.

TABLE 3-1   **BMI Ranges and GLP-1 Medications**

BMI Category	BMI Range	FDA-Approved GLP-1 Medications
Overweight	25.0 to 29.9	Not typically approved unless you have other health issues
Obesity Class I	30.0 to 34.9	Wegovy, Saxenda, Zepbound
Obesity Class II	35.0 to 39.9	Wegovy, Saxenda, Zepbound
Obesity Class III	40.0 or more	Wegovy, Saxenda, Zepbound

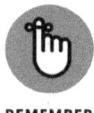

REMEMBER

If you also have type 2 diabetes, medications like Ozempic or Mounjaro might be considered (see Chapter 2 for more details).

Evaluating existing health conditions

Before starting weight-loss medication, your provider will take time to really understand your full health profile. You're not just a BMI number. Tools like the Edmonton Obesity Staging System (EOSS) can help assess how excess weight is affecting your body and quality of life. This can help distinguish whether you have no complications at all from the more severe health issues created by obesity. This kind of staging is often more helpful than BMI alone.

The Edmonton Obesity Staging System (EOSS) assigns a stage from 0 to 4.

>> **Stage 0** means there are no obesity-related health problems yet, so care focuses on identifying contributing factors and supporting healthy eating and physical activity.

>> **Stage 1** involves early risk factors or mild symptoms, where more structured lifestyle changes and closer monitoring are recommended.

>> **Stage 2** occurs when obesity-related medical conditions are present, and doctors may recommend active obesity treatment, including behavioral therapy, medications, or even surgery, while closely managing related health conditions.

>> **Stage 3** reflects more severe health impacts or functional limitations, requiring increasingly intensive treatment.

>> **Stage 4** occurs after you progress through Stage 3 and have uncontrolled complications from obesity despite aggressive management with medicines. In this stage you can experience a wide variety of medical complications, and additional support such as pain management, physical or occupational therapy, and mental health or social support is indicated.

TIP

You might also be asked to complete a STOP-BANG Questionnaire to screen for obstructive sleep apnea (OSA). This is important because sleep apnea is common in people with obesity, and it can impact your safety and outcomes on treatment.

Here are a few other conditions your provider should screen for before prescribing a GLP-RA:

>> High blood pressure

>> Type 2 diabetes or prediabetes

>> High cholesterol

>> Polycystic ovarian syndrome (PCOS)

» Osteoarthritis or mobility issues

» Cardiovascular disease

If you're living with any of these weight-related health conditions, it may make a stronger case for trying a GLP-RA medication. Some GLP-RA drugs have been shown not only to help with weight loss, but also to lower the risk of serious health problems linked to obesity. For example, certain medications such as injectable semaglutide, oral semaglutide (Rybelsus), and injectable dulaglutide (Trulicity) have FDA approval to reduce the risk of major heart-related events like heart attacks and strokes in people with known heart disease, and to help protect kidney function in people with chronic kidney disease.

Understanding the Risks

GLP-1 medications have helped many people, but like all treatments, they're not without risks. Chapter 8 offers you a step-by-step approach for handling drug side effects and other challenges. But before you begin with GLP-1s, you need to possible nutrient deficiencies as well as risks with your doctor. You can find more information about building a care team, including a physician, in Chapter 4.

Noting potential nutrient deficiencies

Using GLP-RA medications can impact vital nutrients your body needs. To be sure you're meeting all recommended daily allowances (RDA), discuss this list and your needs with your provider:

» **Vitamin B12 deficiency:** If you've been on metformin, a common drug prescribed for type 2 diabetes patients, your B12 levels might be low, which, especially for long-term users, can put you at risk for anemia and neurological complications. This risk is not caused by GLP-based weight-loss medications themselves, but it is relevant because many people taking GLP-RAs also have diabetes or insulin resistance and may already be on metformin. Low B12 levels can increase the risk of anemia, nerve problems, and fatigue, which can be mistaken for medication side effects. A simple blood test can check your levels, and you can discuss taking a B12 supplement with your doctor, if necessary.

>> **Iron deficiency:** The GLP-RA medicines can slow stomach emptying and decrease stomach acid production which may lessen your body's ability to absorb iron. Talk to your doctor about monitoring ferritin and considering iron supplementation, particularly if you belong to an at-risk group like menstruating women.

>> **Folate deficiency:** Changes in gut function and lower intake of folate-rich foods may put you at risk for a folate deficiency. Because a daily dose of folate may help support new cell creation and overall health, especially in women of childbearing age, discuss your needs and concerns about folate with your doctor.

>> **Vitamin D and calcium deficiency:** Especially if you're older, weight loss can put your bones at risk. Ask whether a bone density scan is appropriate. Because rapid weight loss and decreased dietary intake can compromise bone health, discuss with your doctor how you can make sure you're getting adequate amounts of calcium and vitamin D to support your bone integrity and metabolism.

>> **Muscle loss:** Fast weight loss can lead to loss of muscle, not just fat. Additionally, GLP-1 agonists like semaglutide and tirzepatide often suppress appetite, which can lead to lower overall protein intake, increased muscle loss if caloric or total protein intake is too low, reduced metabolic rate, and long-term weight regain. Research shows that higher protein diets during weight loss help preserve fat-free mass, especially when combined with resistance exercise. So be sure to eat enough protein and include resistance training in your routine. (See Chapter 5 for exercise regimen and lifestyle suggestions to prevent muscle loss.)

TIP

The recommended protein intake for adults on GLP-1s to lose weight but preserve muscle is 1.2 to 1.5 g/kg of ideal body weight per day. This strategy helps you to preserve lean muscle mass during calorie restriction. This is particularly important if you're over age 50, physically active, or losing weight rapidly.

Example: If your ideal body weight is 70 kg (154 pounds), your target protein intake would be 84 to 105 grams per day:

- 1.2 g/kg × 70 kg = 84 grams/day
- 1.5 g/kg × 70 kg = 105 grams/day

For an overview of typical nutrient recommendations to discuss with your doctor, see Table 3-2.

TABLE 3-2   ## Nutrient Recommendations on GLP-1s

Nutrient	Importance When on GLP-1s	Typical Recommendation
Vitamin B12	Risk of deficiency due to impaired absorption	500 to 1,000 microgram/day
Iron	Reduced acid and intake may impair absorption	Monitor ferritin; supplement as needed
Calcium and vitamin D	Support bone health during weight loss	Ensure RDA-level intake
Folate (B9)	Gut changes and restrictive intake may lower levels	400 to 800 microgram/day
Protein	Preserve lean mass and metabolic function	Adults on GLP-1 therapy

1.2 to 1.5 g/kg of ideal body weight/day or 1.6 to 2.0 g/kg per day for active or older adults

SUPPLEMENTING YOUR CALCIUM AND VITAMIN D WHILE ON GLP-RA MEDICINES

Bone integrity can be compromised on GLP-RAs if you're not getting enough calcium and vitamin D. Keep these tips in mind when discussing calcium and vitamin D supplementation with your doctor.

Because calcium is best absorbed in doses around 500 to 600 mg at a time, you should consider splitting your total daily calcium supplement goal into multiple doses per day. For vitamin D supplementation, you should consider 800–2,000 IU/day of vitamin D_3 (cholecalciferol) while on GLP Ras. While you may encounter higher doses up to 4,000 IU/day, this practice is generally recognized as safe for maintenance in those with low baseline levels, but only when you are under strict medical supervision.

If you are deficient of vitamin D (based on blood work), then you could discuss this common correction regimen with your doctor: Take 50,000 IU weekly for six to eight weeks, and then 1,000 to 2,000 IU/day as maintenance. You should always request your provider check vitamin D levels before starting high-dose supplementation, especially if you're combining it with calcium or have kidney issues. This table offers some general guidelines.

Status	Vitamin D Recommendation	Calcium Recommendation
General maintenance (no deficiency)	800 to 2,000 IU/day	1,000 to 1,200 mg/day (diet and supplements combined)
Obesity, low sun exposure, or on GLP-1	1,000 to 2,000 IU/day (higher doses only under medical supervision)	1,200 mg/day (ensure dietary intake is adequate)

Status	Vitamin D Recommendation	Calcium Recommendation
Vitamin D deficiency (less than 20 ng/mL)	50,000 IU/week for 6 to 8 weeks then maintenance dose	Same as above; do not exceed 2,000 mg/day total
Older adults (over 50 years old)	1,000 to 2,000 IU/day	1,200 mg/day (split dose for better absorption)
Postmenopausal women or at-risk for osteoporosis	1,000 to 2,000 IU/day	1,200 to 1,500 mg/day, under guidance

Realizing additional risks of GLP-RAs

In addition to influencing how your body absorbs and uses certain nutrients, GLP-based medications carry some broader medical risks to be aware of. These are different from the common side effects like nausea or constipation that many people experience early on and learn to manage (see Chapter 8 for more on side effects and tips for handling them). While the overall risk remains low for most patients, doctors should monitor you for the following potential concerns when prescribing you GLP medications:

>> **Thyroid cancer risk:** Before starting a GLP-RA medication, it's important to know that these drugs carry a rare but serious risk of a specific type of thyroid cancer called medullary thyroid carcinoma (MTC). They are not recommended if you have a personal or family history of MTC or a condition called multiple endocrine neoplasia syndrome type 2 (MEN2). If you're unsure about your family history or past diagnoses, please discuss this with your healthcare provider before beginning treatment.

>> **GI side effects:** Nausea, vomiting, or constipation are common, especially early on. These usually get better with time but should be reported to your medical team if they persist. (See Chapter 8 for strategies to manage these side effects.)

>> **Eating disorders or emotional triggers:** If you've had disordered eating in the past, be honest with your care team. GLP-RAs can powerfully suppress appetite and may need extra monitoring by you and your medical team in this case.

>> **Potential weight gain when you stop:** GLP-RAs often need to be taken long-term. If you stop, the weight can return. That's why pairing medication with sustainable lifestyle changes is key.

Detaining the risks is not meant to scare you away from treatment, but to help you make an informed, confident decision. For many people, the health risks of untreated obesity outweigh the potential risks of medication, especially when these medications are used thoughtfully and monitored closely. The key is partnership: having open conversations with your doctor, understanding what to watch for, and using the strategies outlined in this chapter and Chapters 5 and 8 to reduce risk and improve tolerability. With the right guidance and support, many people find these medications to be a safe and effective tool on their weight-loss journey.

Getting Appropriate Tests and Screening

Before you take your first dose, your care team should order labs and other screening tests to make sure it's safe to begin. These tests help identify things like existing nutrient deficiencies, blood sugar issues, or liver and kidney concerns that could affect how well you tolerate the medication (see "Noting potential nutrient deficiencies" for more detail).

These tests also give your team a baseline for tracking progress. Ongoing monitoring is part of using these medications safely and successfully. Periodic check-ins and repeat labs allow your care team to catch problems early, adjust dosing, and address nutrient needs as your eating patterns change. This kind of maintenance helps protect your health while maximizing the benefits of treatment over time.

Expect to take tests like:

>> **A1C and fasting glucose:** These tests show how high your blood sugar runs, both on a day-to-day basis and over the past few months. They help identify diabetes or prediabetes and show how well your body is handling sugar as you lose weight. Because GLP medications can significantly improve blood sugar control, these tests are usually repeated every few months to make sure levels are improving safely and not dropping too low.

>> **Lipid panel:** This test measures different types of cholesterol and fats in your blood that affect heart health. Weight loss and GLP-RA medications often improve cholesterol levels, but changes do not happen overnight. Repeating this test over time helps your doctor track improvements and decide whether other heart-protective treatments are still needed.

>> **Liver:** These blood tests look for signs of liver stress or inflammation. Many people with obesity have fatty liver disease, which often improves with weight

loss, but rapid weight changes can also affect the liver. Periodic testing helps ensure your liver is responding positively as treatment continues.

>> **Kidney function:** These tests measure how well your kidneys are filtering waste from your blood. Good kidney function is important for medication safety, especially as your body size and hydration needs change with your weight loss. Repeat testing helps to confirm that your kidneys are tolerating the medication and lifestyle changes well.

>> **Thyroid panel:** These tests check how well your thyroid gland is working, which affects metabolism, energy, and weight regulation. Thyroid problems can make weight loss harder and may cause symptoms that overlap with medication side effects, such as fatigue or temperature sensitivity. Testing helps rule out thyroid issues before treatment and monitor for changes if symptoms arise.

>> **Vitamin B12, D, iron studies, and folate:** These tests look for deficiencies that can develop when appetite decreases and food intake changes. Low levels can cause fatigue, weakness, hair loss, or nerve symptoms that may be mistaken for medication side effects. Checking these levels at baseline and periodically during treatment allows your doctor to correct deficiencies early and keep you feeling well.

In some cases, your provider might also recommend an EKG or a DEXA scan (for body composition or bone density).

You can review Table 3-3 with your provider to make sure your team makes the right decision on what tests should be ordered to support your personalized needs. Although you'll take all of these tests before you start your meds, you will have to continue taking some at regular intervals to monitor your health.

TABLE 3-3   **Screenings Needed for GLP Medications**

Lab Test	Importance	When to Check
A1C and fasting glucose	Assess glycemic control and diabetes status	Baseline then every 3 to 6 months
Lipid panel	Evaluate cardiovascular risk	Baseline then annually
Comprehensive metabolic panel or hepatic function panel for liver function tests (LFTs)	Check for preexisting liver issues	Baseline, then if clinically indicated
Renal function pane or basic metabolic panel for electrolytes and kidney function (creatinine, eGFR)	To check for dehydration-related changes	Baseline, then at least annually

(continued)

TABLE 3-3 *(continued)*

Lab Test	Importance	When to Check
Thyroid stimulating hormone (TSH) and free T4	For thyroid function, especially if family history of thyroid disease or nodules present	Baseline (optional) then only if symptoms arise
Vitamin B12	Risk if also on metformin	Baseline then every 1 to 2 years if at risk
Vitamin D and calcium	Monitor for bone health, especially during rapid weight loss	Baseline then every 6 to 12 months if at risk
Iron studies (ferritin, iron, TIBC)	Appetite suppression may reduce iron intake	Baseline then repeat if have symptoms or at risk

Finding GLP Medications on Alternative Platforms

Most people start their weight-loss journey by working with a primary care clinician or a dedicated weight-management team who can provide in-depth evaluation, ongoing monitoring, and personalized guidance (for more info on your healthcare team, see Chapter 4). Some patients, however, turn to consumer telehealth platforms as another way to access weight-loss medications, especially when local care is limited or hard to schedule.

TIP

These platforms typically offer online questionnaires and virtual visits that can lead to a prescription for GLP-based or other weight-loss medications. While they can be convenient and improve access, they may not always provide the same level of comprehensive care outlined earlier in this chapter, such as detailed lab monitoring, long-term follow-up, or coordinated nutrition and lifestyle support. For this reason, these services are best viewed as access points, not full replacements for a medical team.

Consumer telehealth platforms, including Hims, Found, Ro, and Whole Health Rx, may be helpful if you live in an area with limited obesity specialists, have difficulty getting timely appointments, or are looking for an initial entry point into treatment. Even when using these platforms, it is still important to involve your regular healthcare provider to ensure appropriate monitoring, lab testing, and long-term safety.

In the following list, we detail some of the most popular and reputable platforms for these medications:

>> **Hims** offers GLP-1 injections and personalized oral medication kits starting at $69 per month (10-month plan), with compounded semaglutide available from $199/month, and it includes app-based tools, meal plans, and anti-nausea support.

>> **Found** charges $99 to $149/month for membership (not including GLP-1s), with injections costing $650 to $1,500/month on top, and average self-reported weight loss is around 12 percent in one year.

>> **Ro** has its Body Program, which includes a discounted fee of $45 for the first month, and then membership cost $145 per month (medication costs separate). Branded GLP-1s range from $349 to $1,700 per month, though some proprietary single-dose vials are priced at $349 to $499.

>> **Whole Health Rx** (offered via Vitamin Shoppe) charges a $219 per month for its subscription covering telehealth access to GLP-1 medications like Ozempic, Mounjaro, and Rybelsus, but this fee likely excludes drug costs and is a newer entrant with much less published user satisfaction data as other platforms.

TIP

Hims balances affordability, convenience, and relatively strong user ratings. Found offers robust support but with higher extra costs. Ro delivers comprehensive care tools but with variable customer experience. Whole Health Rx appears promising for GLP-1 access, though the information for you to review patient feedback online is still limited.

2

Using Weight-Loss Medications Healthfully

Discover how to partner with your healthcare provider to use weight-loss medications safely and effectively.

See what to expect at your first visit, how clinicians screen for medical risks, and the steps they take when choosing or adjusting a medication.

Uncover how lifestyle habits like nutrition, movement, sleep, and stress management work alongside medication to improve results and protect your health.

Understand how to track progress, manage side effects, and build long-term routines that help keep the weight off once you've lost it.

Chapter **4**

Seeking Healthcare Guidance

When it comes to losing weight in a healthy, sustainable way you do not have to go it alone. To be successful, having a team surround you with support increases your chances of success. After all, your goal isn't just to drop a few pounds and call it quits.

Because we want you to feel better, reduce health risks, and build habits you can sustain forever, this chapter gives you the info you need to assemble your team a team that can help you establish your plan and give you the support you need. In this chapter, we tell you how to choose your team, what roles each member plays, how often you should meet, and how prescriptions and insurance fit into the overall picture.

Establishing Your Care Team

Consider what it means to have a care team. You might think of needing a doctor, coach, trainer, nutritionist, or all of the above. Although your physician is key to your team, others can help you manage specific points of your care with specialized information. For example, a nutrition coach can support your unique nutritional needs while a trainer can help guide your exercise plan. These people might all work in the same clinic, or you may assemble them separately. But what matters is gathering the right support. These sections help you understand the roles of each person you can add to your team so you can assemble a group of pros to support your specific needs.

Finding the right fit for your physician

Your physician is the quarterback of your weight-loss team. They help decide when medication is appropriate, choose the safest option based on your medical history, and adjust the plan as your body responds. Your physician also serves as the central hub of communication, coordinating lab work, monitoring you for risks and side effects, and making sure guidance from dietitians, pharmacists, and other specialists fits together into one clear plan. In short, they help "call the plays" so your treatment stays safe, effective, and aligned with your long-term health goals.

So you want a doctor who has some additional training in obesity medicine. So you should narrow down the list of possibilities first by making sure the doctors you have in mind are board certified in obesity medicine.

TIP

To find out if your physician is board certified in obesity medicine (a Diplomat of the American Board of Obesity Medicine [DABOM]), start by visiting the American Board of Obesity Medicine's website and use their public "Find a Physician" search tool at https://abom.learningbuilder.com/Search/Public/MemberRole/CertificationVerification. With this tool, you can enter the doctor's name or location to confirm active certification status. If you're unsure, you can also ask your doctor directly. Just because a clinician prescribes GLP-RAs does not make them an obesity medicine specialist.

TIP

Finding the right doctor for weight-loss care does not have to mean cycling through multiple appointments that feel uncomfortable or discouraging. A good starting point is to look for clinicians who explicitly list obesity medicine, metabolic health, or weight management as an area of focus on their website or professional profile. Board certification in obesity medicine, endocrinology, or internal medicine, as well as experience prescribing GLP-RA medications, can signal that a provider is familiar with current, evidence-based approaches.

It can be helpful to ask a few targeted questions before scheduling or during your first visit to see if a doctor is the right fit for you. You can ask things like:

>> How do you view obesity — as a chronic medical condition or a lifestyle issue?

>> What is your experience prescribing and monitoring weight-loss medications like GLP-1s and other GLP-RAs?

>> How do you approach long-term treatment and follow-up, including lab monitoring and dose adjustments?

>> Do you work with or refer to dietitians, pharmacists, or other specialists as part of your obesity care model?

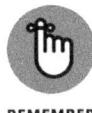

REMEMBER

Pay attention not just to the answers, but to how you feel during the conversation. A good fit is a provider who listens without judgment, explains options clearly, and includes you in decision-making rather than rushing you into or away from medication. If your primary care provider is supportive but not experienced with weight-loss medications, asking for a referral to a specialist can be a helpful next step instead of starting over on your own. Your relationship with your clinician is key. If you don't feel heard or supported, it's okay to look for another one.

Considering coaches you might need

When it comes to coaching for weight loss, four key areas make the biggest impact: nutrition, lifestyle, exercise, and behavioral health. Despite recent encouraging results with AI coaches, traditional, human coaches are the mainstay of this treatment option, at least for now.

The different types of coaching you might want to use include these following types:

>> **Nutrition coaching** focuses on building balanced eating habits and calorie awareness. When it comes to weight loss, food is your foundation. Studies show that a calorie deficit is required for weight loss, and dietary interventions are the cornerstone of any weight-loss plan. So working with a nutrition coach or dietitian helps you tailor what you eat so it fits your life and culture rather than copying someone else's plan.

>> **Lifestyle coaching** helps identify daily patterns like sleep, stress, and routine; research links better sleep and lower stress with improved long-term weight management. A plan that includes lifestyle changes along with diet and exercise is more successful. Ask your team about small changes that you can keep make and maintain for years. You should leave each session with one to two concrete action steps, not just "try harder next week."

>> **Exercise coaching** keeps you accountable and helps you find enjoyable physical activities, which studies show improves adherence and doubles the chance of sustained weight loss over a year. Movement matters. Both aerobic and resistance exercise help build muscle, boost metabolism, and improve health beyond just losing weight. How do you know if your coach is legit? You are probably reading a theme by now, qualifications matter!

>> **Behavioral health coaching** focuses on mindset and emotional triggers. Weight-loss programs integrated with behavioral therapy elements lead to 3 to 5 percent more weight loss on average. Your mindset matters, and behavior-change counseling, self-monitoring, goal setting, and support groups can help you succeed. Don't skip this piece.

TIP

You can find the right coaches by following these tips:

>> **When choosing a nutrition professional,** credentials matter: Look for a Registered Dietitian (RD or RDN), not just a self-described "nutrition coach." Studies show that people who work with a registered dietitian lose significantly more weight than those who try on their own. You can find a good fit online at www.eatright.org.

>> **When choosing a lifestyle coach,** remember that anyone can call themselves a "health coach." Ask about their training. Teammates who completed programs certified by the National Board for Health & Wellness Coaching (NBHWC) are the gold standard. You can search for great options at https://www.joincalibrate.com/lp/coaching-and-curriculum.

>> **When choosing an exercise coach,** look for certifications like NASM, ACSM, or NSCA. Bonus points if your exercise coach has worked with clients managing obesity or chronic health conditions in the past. Your coach should help you find something you enjoy so that you will stick with it. Look at www.acefitness.org or www.nasm.org to check out some good options.

>> **When choosing a behavioral health coach,** two potentially helpful credentials would be either LCSW or PsyD. An LCSW is a Licensed Clinical Social Worker, and a PsyD is a Doctor of Psychology. Both are advanced mental health professionals, but they differ in training and focus. Searching on www.psychologytoday.com will pair you with a great match.

REMEMBER

Don't be afraid to "shop around," but know that you can often narrow the field before ever stepping into an exam room. Reading provider bios, looking for stated experience in obesity or metabolic care, and asking targeted screening questions in advance can help you identify a better fit from the start. While it's normal to try one or two providers, finding someone whose approach aligns with your needs can make a real difference, because a strong therapeutic relationship is one of the most powerful predictors of long-term success.

LETTING AI WEIGH IN ON YOUR WEIGHT-LOSS GOALS

AI is emerging as a new coach in the weight-loss realm. A recent study showed that AI-based lifestyle coaching performed just as well as traditional human-led programs for people with pre-diabetes and obesity. The AI program used automated nudges based on reinforcement learning instead of live coaches or group sessions. Both the AI and human programs achieved meaningful weight loss and improvements in activity or HbA1c. Interestingly, the AI program had higher participation and completion rates.

Several AI tools can be useful for weight-loss support, especially when used alongside medical care. General-purpose AI platforms like ChatGPT, Google Gemini, and Microsoft Copilot can help with meal planning, habit building, and problem-solving around daily challenges. Nutrition-focused apps that use AI, such as MyFitnessPal, Lose It!, or Cronometer, are especially helpful for tracking food intake and spotting patterns over time. The best choice depends on whether you want conversational coaching, structured tracking, or a mix of both.

AI tends to work best when you use it actively and consistently. Helpful ways to use AI for weight loss include:

- **Taking photos of meals** and asking AI or an app to estimate calories or portion sizes and suggest adjustments

- **Creating simple meal plans** for the week, then generating a grocery list that fits your preferences, budget, or time constraints

- **Planning ahead for challenges,** such as asking for strategies for eating out, traveling, or managing cravings in the evening

- **Daily or weekly check-ins,** where you ask AI to help you reflect on what went well and what to adjust next

- **Habit building support,** such as reminders to hydrate, move, or eat protein earlier in the day

- **Recipe swaps,** where you ask for lighter versions of favorite meals that still feel satisfying

Used thoughtfully, AI can act like a steady, judgment-free assistant that helps you stay organized and motivated between doctor visits, while your healthcare team continues to guide medical decisions.

Setting visit frequency

Frequent contact with your doctor and long-term follow-up are linked to better weight-loss outcomes. Your doctor typically helps set the visit schedule, but it's something you can and should discuss together based on your needs and preferences. Early on, especially during the dose escalation period when medication doses are slowly increased over the first three months, visits are often scheduled every four to six weeks to check progress, manage side effects, and adjust dosing. After you reach a stable maintenance dose, follow-up visits are usually spaced out to every three to six months.

These appointments are about more than the number on the scale. Your care team may order lab work during some visits to monitor things like blood sugar, cholesterol, kidney function, or nutrient levels, helping ensure that weight loss is happening safely and supporting your overall health (see Chapter 3 for more on lab monitoring).

In addition to physician follow-up, meeting regularly with coaches or support staff can further improve results and make a meaningful difference, especially early in treatment. During the first one to two months, many programs recommend weekly visits, when routines are being established and medication doses are often changing. These early sessions typically focus on practical topics like managing early side effects, building simple meals that work with reduced appetite, setting realistic movement goals, and troubleshooting common challenges.

From months three to six, visits may continue weekly or shift to every other week, depending on your needs and progress. These sessions are often used to fine-tune nutrition, adjust activity plans, reinforce habits, and maintain motivation as weight loss continues. After this initial phase, follow-up may become less frequent, but ongoing support remains important for sustaining progress and long-term success. You can learn more about tracking progress and monitoring weight loss in Chapter 6.

TIP

If you feel overwhelmed with the idea of all these visits to doctors and coaches, don't worry. We put together with a suggested follow-up protocol in Table 4-1 so you have a roadmap to follow. Discuss this with your doctor and make adjustments based on their advice and your unique needs.

WARNING

Don't skip your check-ins if you're serious about losing weight. No one is trying to sell you a vacation condo, give you a guilt trip, or trap you into anything during these visits. Your team is doing the opposite: trying to empower you and set you free. These visits help reinforce the boundaries you've created together and motivate you to keep going. Even after you feel and see huge results, you might think skipping check-ins won't hurt, but it's easy to slip into old habits. So to keep yourself on track and to make changes that really stick, let your team decide how frequently you should meet and when you're really to let go.

TABLE 4-1 Team Follow-Up Frequency

Phase	Doctor Visits	Coaching Check-Ins
Months 1 to 3 (dose escalation period)	One visit per month	Weekly
Months 4 to 12	One visit every 3 months	Monthly
Months 12 and beyond	Every 3 or 6 months as suggested by your physician	As needed for support

Getting and Paying for Your Prescription

You've arrived at a key step in the process: getting your medication in hand. Beyond receiving a prescription, getting these medications often involves navigating insurance coverage, prior authorizations, pharmacy availability, and out-of-pocket costs. This process can feel confusing or frustrating, but it's a common part of treatment and something your care team can help you manage. These sections help you understand some of the details better.

Choosing the best route to fill your prescription

You have several options for filling your weight-loss medication prescription, and the best choice often depends on your insurance, location, cost considerations, and how much medical support you want. Many people think first of a local pharmacy, but prescriptions can be obtained and filled through several routes, each with different benefits.

>> **Your regular clinic:** This route offers continuity and coordination of care, since your doctor already knows your medical history and can easily order labs and follow up. Prescriptions are often sent to familiar retail or health-system pharmacies such as CVS, Walgreens, or Kaiser Permanente pharmacies, which can simplify insurance coverage and refills.

>> **A specialist:** Specialists often have deeper experience with GLP-1 medications and complex cases. Clinics affiliated with academic centers or specialty groups, such as obesity medicine clinics, endocrinology practices, or metabolic health centers (for example, programs within Mayo Clinic, Cleveland Clinic, or large university health systems), may be especially helpful if you have multiple health conditions or prior medication challenges.

>> **Telehealth (online pharmacy):** Telehealth services can offer faster access and convenience, particularly if local providers are limited. Well-known

platforms that provide weight-loss care include Hims, Found, Ro, or Whole Health Rx. These companies are discussed in more detail in Chapter 3.

>> **Mail-order pharmacy:** Mail-order pharmacies deliver medications directly to your home and are commonly used for ongoing treatment. Large, reputable options include Express Scripts, CVS Caremark, and OptumRx, which are often tied to insurance plans and may offer cost savings. Because GLP-1 medications are temperature-sensitive, it's important to ensure any mail-order pharmacy follows proper cold-shipping standards.

Knowing these options helps you compare convenience, cost, and level of support, and it sets the stage for understanding how to choose a safe, legitimate pharmacy as you move forward.

TIP

Regardless of what route you take, make sure you're getting your prescriptions filled from safe pharmacy, especially when ordering online. Always follow the FDA's recommendations for procuring medicines through online pharmacies (`https://www.fda.gov/drugs/besaferx-your-source-online-pharmacy-information/considering-online-pharmacy`).

Look for these signs that a pharmacy operates safely and legally. Safe pharmacies always

>> Require a doctor's prescription and have a clear U.S. address and phone number

>> Employ a licensed pharmacist to answer questions and are registered with a state board of pharmacy

>> Follow good manufacturing practices and meet Pharmacy Compounding Accreditation Board (PCAB) and National Association of Boards of Pharmacy (NABP) accreditation standards, if compounding medications

WARNING

Warning signs include not requiring a prescription, hiding license information, or lacking a pharmacist to consult. Be cautious if the medicine arrives damaged or looks different from what you'd get locally and avoid any company that doesn't clearly protect your personal and financial information, as these are major red flags for unsafe or counterfeit operations.

When figuring out which source is best for you, consider these factors:

>> **Convenience:** How easy it is to get and stay on your medication matters. This includes how quickly the pharmacy can fill your prescription, whether you can pick it up locally or have it delivered to your home, and how simple refills are to manage. For many people, convenience also means fewer phone calls,

shorter wait times, and less back-and-forth when doses change during the dose-escalation period.

>> **Cost:** Price is often the biggest deciding factor. Insurance coverage, copays, deductibles, manufacturer savings cards, and whether a pharmacy accepts your insurance all influence out-of-pocket costs. Some people choose mail-order or specialty pharmacies because they are less expensive, while others pay more at retail pharmacies for faster access or in-person support.

>> **Safety:** Weight-loss medications, especially injectable GLP-1s, require proper storage, handling, and dosing. Reputable pharmacies follow strict temperature controls, provide clear instructions, and verify prescriptions directly with your doctor. Safety also includes knowing that the medication is FDA-approved, correctly labeled, and dispensed by a licensed pharmacy.

>> **Access and availability:** Supply shortages can affect where people fill prescriptions. Some pharmacies have more reliable access to certain medications or doses, which may influence your choice, especially early in treatment when timing matters.

>> **Level of support:** Some pharmacies and telehealth platforms offer extra help, such as medication education, injection training, refill reminders, or access to pharmacists who can answer questions. This added support can be especially helpful when you are just starting treatment or adjusting doses.

>> **Coordination with your care team:** Pharmacies that communicate easily with your doctor can streamline prior authorizations, dose changes, and lab requirements. Strong coordination reduces delays and frustration and helps keep your treatment on track.

THE PEARLS AND PITFALLS OF ONLINE TELEHEALTH COMPANIES

Online telehealth companies have made it easier to access weight-loss medications and coaching from home. Convenience is a major draw, especially for busy people who want fast access to treatment. But not all telehealth services are created equal, and it is important to know what to look for. Make sure any company you use employs licensed, board-certified providers and requires a real medical evaluation before prescribing medication. Some programs such as Found, Calibrate, and Sequence offer physician oversight, lab testing, and ongoing support for nutrition and lifestyle.

- Found presents itself as a telehealth weight-care platform that combines clinical oversight with personalized lifestyle and medication support. It emphasizes access

(continued)

(continued)

and scalability, with the claim that its virtual model makes obesity care more afford-able and reachable. Found points out that its services are now covered by major U.S. health insurance plans, broadening access.

- Calibrate's mission is to "change the way the world treats weight" by focusing on metabolic health rather than willpower alone. It combines clinician-prescribed GLP-1 medications with one-on-one video coaching and a structured curriculum across food, sleep, exercise and emotional health. The program claims average weight losses of around 16 to 19 percent over the first one to three years.

- Sequence is positioned as a telehealth subscription platform (now part of WW/WeightWatchers) that offers access to healthcare providers who can prescribe weight-loss medications (like GLP-1s) and combine that with diet/behavioral sup-port. It claims to simplify insurance coordination and provide a digital first-model for chronic weight management.

Be cautious of sites that promise quick results or ship drugs without verifying your health history. Read reviews, check refund policies, and confirm that prescriptions come from legitimate U.S. pharmacies. The best telehealth programs include follow-up visits, lab monitoring, and access to nutrition or behavioral support. A smart con-sumer asks questions, compares options, and only partners with services that value safety as much as convenience. Chapter 3 gives you the details of various consumer telehealth platforms that offer access specifically for weight-loss medication, such as Hims, Found, Ro, and Whole Health Rx.

Getting the best deal on weight-loss meds

To get the best deal on weight-loss medications, start by comparing pharmacy prices with tools like GoodRx or SingleCare. GoodRx and SingleCare both help patients access lower cash prices for prescription medications, but they differ in how they source and present those discounts:

>> **GoodRx** (https://www.goodrx.com) aggregates pricing data from multiple pharmacy benefit managers (PBMs), pharmacy chains, and discount networks, which often results in a wider range of coupon options for a single drug. GoodRx frequently shows multiple competing coupon prices for comparison and also provides additional features like medication-tracking tools and price-change alerts.

>> **SingleCare** (https://www.singlecare.com), on the other hand, partners directly with pharmacies and PBMs to negotiate fixed discounted cash prices, which can sometimes be lower but may be available at fewer locations. SingleCare typically highlights one negotiated rate per pharmacy and focuses more on simplified coupon access without requiring an account.

TIP

Both tools can significantly reduce out-of-pocket costs, but the better option often depends on your preferred pharmacy and the specific medication being purchased.

You can also use these tips to get the best deal on your meds:

>> Check manufacturer websites for savings cards or patient-assistance programs that can lower costs.

>> See whether mail-order or specialty pharmacies offer discounts on bulk fills or negotiated copays.

>> Consider compounded medications only from licensed pharmacies using FDA-approved ingredients.

>> Ask your doctor about switching to lower-cost alternatives in the same class. If insurance denies coverage, file an appeal with supporting medical documentation.

>> Request samples or starter doses from your provider to cut down on or bridge early costs.

>> Watch for market changes when new drugs launch or prices drop.

WARNING

Avoid unverified online sellers to protect both your health and your wallet. A verified online pharmacy requires a valid prescription, is licensed in the United States, and clearly lists a physical address and licensed pharmacist. Legitimate pharmacies also source FDA-approved medications, follow proper storage and shipping standards, and provide contact information if you have questions or concerns.

TIP

Here are the top three red flags that signal an unsafe or unverified online seller:

>> **No prescription required:** If a website offers weight-loss medications without requiring a valid prescription from a licensed clinician, it is not operating safely or legally.

>> **Unclear licensing or contact information:** Legitimate pharmacies clearly list a U.S. address, pharmacy license, and a way to contact a licensed pharmacist. Missing or vague contact details are a major warning sign.

>> **Prices or claims that seem too good to be true:** Extremely low prices, guaranteed results, or language that downplays risks and side effects often indicate counterfeit, diluted, or improperly handled products.

Navigating Health Insurance Coverage for Obesity

Navigating health insurance coverage for obesity can feel frustrating, but understanding a few basics helps. Many insurance plans now recognize obesity as a chronic disease, which means they may cover treatments like nutrition counseling, behavioral therapy, medications, or even bariatric surgery. Coverage often depends on your body mass index (BMI) and whether you have related health conditions such as diabetes or high blood pressure.

In many cases, your insurer requires prior authorization, meaning your doctor must submit documentation explaining why the treatment is medically necessary before the medication is approved. Sometimes, despite doing everything right, you may receive a letter from your insurance company denying coverage. If this happens, your first step should be to call the insurer and ask for a clear explanation of *why* the medication was denied and what additional information is needed. This is where taking notes helps. You need to ask specific questions about what's covered, what documentation is required, and what copays or limits apply Ask whether the denial is due to missing documentation, step-therapy requirements (trying another medication first), or plan exclusions (for example, your insurer does not cover this medication and requests your doctor to select an alternative).

Next, contact the right person at your doctor's office to help move the process forward. This is usually not your doctor or the front desk staff, but someone who works directly with insurance companies, such as a prior authorization specialist, billing coordinator, insurance navigator, or office nurse manager. Share the denial details and ask them to submit an appeal or additional paperwork on your behalf. Appeals often involve resubmitting records, adding supporting diagnoses, or writing a medical necessity letter, and many approvals happen at this stage.

TIP

No matter who you call, ask specific questions about what's covered, what documentation is required, and what copays or limits apply. You can make taking notes even easier by using an AI scribe during the phone call. Free or low-cost AI tools can listen in on your phone calls or meetings and take notes for you. Staying organized and persistent usually pays off when it comes to getting obesity care covered.

If something is denied, ask your doctor's office to help with appeals.

CULLING COSTS BY STREAMLINING ACCESS TO GLP-RA MEDS

As demand for weight-loss medications surges, so have prices. This has created cost barriers for many who might benefit. The World Health Organization recently signaled support for using GLP-RA drugs globally, but noted that current costs, often over $1,000 dollars per month, restrict access. However, direct-pay models between patients and manufacturers are emerging as the real disruptor in this economic space that may bring costs down.

Lilly's agreement with the U.S. government to expand access through LillyDirect is highlighted as an example of getting your meds straight from the source. This model may represent the future of obesity medicine distribution. Such a break-through pricing deal in the U.S., announced by Donald Trump and major manufac-turers in 2025, aims to cut monthly costs. In exchange for giving patients direct access, manufacturers are granted tariff protection and fast-track FDA review as part of the deal.

Medicare coverage has also expanded to include several obesity-related medica-tions, with copays capped at $50 per month for insured patients and costs for uninsured/self-pay patients as low as $149 dollars per month. Together these developments suggest a transformation in how weight-loss treatments are priced and covered.

Bottom line: Consumers may soon get access to powerful therapies at a much lower cost, but it remains important to check and confirm what your plan actually covers to protect your weight-loss investment.

Understanding Prescribing Protocols

When starting GLP-RAs or similar weight-loss medications, doctors follow a gradual, structured approach to help your body adjust to the drug. This approach is designed to reduce any side effects you may experience. These sections break down the protocols for both brand-name drugs as well as compounded versions so you have an idea of what your path may look like. Discuss these protocols with your doctor so that you know exactly what you'll experience and how and when you might adjust.

Getting a handle on brand-name dosing practices

Your doctor will be with you every step of the way for your treatments so tha you are completely supported to manage side effects and adjust gradually to your medication. A typical path your doctor will follow looks like this:

>> **Low starting dose:** Treatment usually begins with a low starting dose to test tolerance and minimize nausea or gastrointestinal upset. This dose will stay constant for several weeks.

>> **Titration period:** After several weeks, the dose is slowly increased (uptitrated) according to manufacturer and guideline schedules until the target mainte-nance dose is reached — the level shown to provide the most effective weight loss while still being well-tolerated. This titration period typically spans eight to sixteen weeks, depending on the drug and how your body responds.

During this time, your healthcare provider checks in regularly to monitor side effects, hydration, blood sugar levels, and progress toward goals. If symptoms like nausea or constipation become bothersome, your doctor may hold the current dose longer or step back to the previous level before resuming upward titration. You should check out a more in-depth walkthrough of managing side effects in Chapter 8.

>> **Continued therapy:** Once the maintenance dose is achieved, you stay at that dose long-term, as continuing therapy is necessary to maintain benefits. Most guidelines say treatment should be ongoing. Once you lose weight you still need support to maintain it.

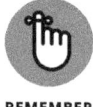

REMEMBER

Stopping treatment too early often leads to regaining weight. This book can give you the keys to being successful in selecting the weight-loss solution that enhances your lifelong term. Even if you meet challenges, this text can serve as your roadmap to success. Long-term treatment will be crucial. For more on this, check out Chapter 9.

In short, prescribing these medicines is a careful, gradual process designed to bal-ance effectiveness, comfort, and safety. Table 4-2 gives you a look at a basic plan followed by most obesity medicine specialists for increasing the dose of your medication gradually until you reach the appropriate maintenance dose.

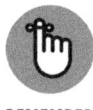

REMEMBER

The gradual doses you're taking allow your body to adjust, but it all depends on what you are prescribed. Your doctor will monitor you and increase doses when nausea is controlled, and they will check-in with you about constipation, heart-burn, and other side effects. Be sure to report any side effects you're experiencing, from fatigue or dizziness to heartburn and nausea, and check out Chapter 8 for more on managing these.

MICRODOSING — A MARKETING TREND

The American Association of Clinical Endocrinology has stated that microdosing GLP-1 medications is not supported by scientific evidence. The organization recommends sticking to FDA-approved dosing guidelines instead. Most data supporting microdosing are anecdotal, and there are no large, randomized trials validating this practice. You should know that some direct-to-consumer weight-loss companies such as Noom have promoted microdosed GLP-1 medications to people with a BMI of 25, despite the lack of medical guidelines supporting this practice. Even when using Noom's "calculator," you technically should not qualify for medication with a BMI slightly above 25 alone in the absence of other risk factor like diabetes. Microdosing may be considered only in rare cases, such as severe side effects or "super responders," but should be managed carefully and individually.

Bottom line: Micro-dosing is a marketing trend, not a medically validated treatment.

TABLE 4-2 ## Typical Dosing Schedule for GLP Medications

Medication (Brand Name)	Starting Dose	Typical Uptitration Frequency	Maintenance Dose
Semaglutide (Wegovy/ Ozempic)	0.25 mg once weekly	Increase every four weeks	2.4 mg once weekly
Tirzepatide (Zepbound/ Mounjaro)	2.5 mg once weekly	Increase every four weeks	15 mg once weekly
Liraglutide (Saxenda)	0.6 mg once daily	Increase weekly	3.0 mg once daily
Dulaglutide (Trulicity)	0.75 mg once weekly	Increase every four weeks	4.5 mg once weekly
Oral Semaglutide (Rybelsus)	3 mg once daily	Every thirty days	14 mg once daily

Exploring common protocols for compounded medications

Recent shortages of brand-name weight-loss drugs have led many people to explore compounded versions of semaglutide and similar medications. Compounding pharmacies make custom formulations that can cost less but may differ in purity and stability from FDA-approved drugs. They also potentially offer alternative drug delivery mechanisms, such as oral tablets, capsules, or drops, if you have a fear of needles. While helping patients afford medication is compassionate, using compounded drugs *purely* to cut costs is generally not allowed.

You should be aware that compounding without medical justification falls outside the regulatory framework that governs prescription medications. The FDA has warned that these products can carry risks like dosing errors or contamination because they are not reviewed for safety or effectiveness.

Common protocols for compounded GLP-1 and weight-loss medications vary by pharmacy and prescriber but generally aim to mimic the dosing patterns of FDA-approved drugs like semaglutide (Ozempic/Wegovy) or tirzepatide (Mounjaro/Zepbound). Here's what clinical practice with a typical compounding pharmacy looks like:

>> **Starting low and titrating slowly:**

- **Compounded GLP-1 regimens:** Most begin with 0.25 mg once weekly and increase every four weeks to 0.5 mg, 1 mg, 1.7 mg, and up to 2.4 mg weekly, depending on tolerance and response.

- **Tirzepatide-based compounds:** Doses often start at 2.5 mg weekly and may increase every 4 weeks up to 10–15 mg as tolerated.

- **Combination formulations:** Some compounders mix GLP-1 analogs with vitamin B12, L-carnitine, or NAD+, though these additions are not standardized and lack clinical trial data.

>> **Monitoring:** Clinicians recommend baseline labs, monthly follow-ups during dose escalation, and continued evaluation every three to six months for safety, side effects, and weight response.

No compounded GLP-1 product has been evaluated or approved by the FDA, and potency, sterility, and stability can vary by source. Professional guidelines advise using FDA-approved formulations whenever possible and considering compounded options only when commercial products are unavailable. The message is that safety and legal compliance must guide decisions, not price alone. The section earlier in this chapter, "Choosing the best route to fill your prescription," covers a range of considerations and safety factors pharmacies, including compounding pharmacies, must follow. Patients should discuss these options with their healthcare provider and use compounded drugs only when FDA-approved versions are unavailable. Check out Chapter 2 for a deeper dive into compounding risks and benefits.

Chapter **5**

Integrating Medications with Lifestyle Changes

G LP-RA medications have transformed how people approach weight loss by regulating hunger, improving insulin sensitivity, and supporting sustained weight reduction. But these medications aren't a magic "pill" for you to use as the sole strategy for your weight loss.

REMEMBER

The most successful, lasting weight transformations happen when you combine medication with intentional changes in nutrition that focus on the quality of food you are eating to ensure that you get all of the nutrients and minerals you need. Physical activity — both movement and strength training — are critical to preserve muscle mass.

In this chapter, you find out about healthy eating choices that offer nutrient-dense foods to fuel your body while you lose weight, as well as the types of supplements that address potential nutritional gaps when consuming fewer calories. You also discover how fitting exercise into your weekly (or daily) routines supports your weight-loss efforts.

Rethinking Nutrition and Diet

When you eat less, you need to eat smarter. Every bite matters. Because you feel fuller more quickly when taking GLP-RA medication, the key for adequate nutrition is to opt for nutrient-dense foods. Nutrient-dense foods are foods that provide a lot of vitamins, minerals, protein, and healthy fats in relatively small portions, such as eggs, fish, lean meats, beans, Greek yogurt, vegetables, fruits, nuts, and whole grains. Choosing these foods helps ensure you get adequate nutrition even when your overall food intake is lower, supporting energy levels, muscle health, and long-term success on medication.

Basic nutrition concepts

When people talk about "macros," they are referring to macronutrients, the nutrients your body needs in larger amounts to function every day. These include carbohydrates, which provide quick energy; protein, which supports muscle, metabolism, and feeling full; and fats, which help with hormone production, brain health, and absorbing certain vitamins. In addition to macros, your body also needs micronutrients, which are vitamins and minerals required in smaller amounts but are just as important for health. Examples of "micros" include vitamins like A, B12, and D, and minerals such as calcium and phosphorus for bones. Sodium is another important mineral that can affect blood pressure and kidney function. When you're eating less, getting the right balance of macros and enough micronutrients becomes especially important. Thinking about nutrition this way helps you choose foods that support your body, not just fill your stomach. You can dive deeper into your specific needs below in the later section, "Creating Balanced, Satisfying Meals."

How to read a food label

A food label helps you understand what you're actually eating and how it fits into your nutritional needs. Start with the serving size, because all the numbers on the label are based on that amount, not the entire package. Next, look at protein, fiber, and added sugars, which are especially important when managing appetite and blood sugar. Finally, check the vitamin and mineral section to see whether the food contributes nutrients like calcium, iron, or potassium, and use this information to compare foods and make more informed choices.

Prioritizing your new nutritional needs

When appetite changes with weight-loss medication, the way you think about food often needs to change, too. Many people were taught to focus on food rules and restrictions or to avoid entire food groups, but those approaches don't always work when you're eating less overall. With GLP–RA medications, the goal shifts from "eating less" to eating with purpose, making sure the food you choose delivers the nutrients your body still needs.

REMEMBER

Because you may feel full quickly, your nutritional priorities become more intentional. Instead of thinking in terms of foods you should cut out, it helps to think about what your body needs first to maintain energy, muscle, bone health, and overall well–being. Reframing food as fuel, rather than something to limit or control, can make eating feel more supportive and less stressful during this process.

Use this list for guidance on how you can reframe your perspective on food:

>> **Prioritize protein** to maintain lean body mass because when you lose weight, you want to lose the fat and keep the muscle.

Protein is critical not just for maintaining muscle, but also for strength, energy, and recovery. It also helps to preserve skin and hair during rapid fat loss. And because carbs are often eaten before protein (think of pasta as a first course) and you become fuller faster on GLP-RAs, protein can often get skipped. Be intentional about protein intake. Good options include eggs, fish, poultry, lean meats, tofu, beans, Greek yogurt, and cottage cheese.

>> **Focus on fiber** to improve gut health and satiety; fiber helps you keep your digestive system working smoothly and regularly and also helps you feel full. This is key because GLP-RAs can slow down digestion. High-fiber choices include beans, lentils, oats, barley, and whole grains.

>> **Include vegetables** for volume and micronutrients and antioxidants with relatively few calories, making them ideal when appetite is reduced. Non-starchy vegetables such as leafy greens, broccoli, cauliflower, peppers, zucchini, and carrots can add volume and nutrients without overwhelming your stomach. Cooking vegetables can also make them easier to tolerate early in treatment.

>> **Choose fruits for nutrients and natural sweetness** provide fiber, vitamins, and hydration, and can help satisfy sweet cravings without relying on added sugars. Options like berries, apples, citrus, pears, and stone fruits are especially helpful because they offer fiber along with natural sweetness. Pairing fruit with protein or fat, such as yogurt or nuts, can improve tolerance and blood sugar control.

>> **Choose nutrient-dense, whole foods** to avoid deficiencies. Dairy or dairy alternatives, nuts, seeds, and whole grains help prevent nutrient deficiencies and support energy, immunity, and long-term health.

When needed, add a dietary supplement to get the levels of vitamins and minerals you need. Check out the later section, "Considering Supplements While Taking GLP-RAs" for more on supplements.

>> **Cut out ultra-processed foods** — Foods that contain artificial ingredients, preservatives, added sugars, or refined starches, or that have been significantly altered from their natural form. Common examples include soft drinks, candy, chips, packaged snack foods, sweetened breakfast cereals, instant soups, frozen entrees, and most commercially packaged breads (especially those with long ingredient lists, added sugars, and dough conditioners).

TIP

In place of processed foods, opt for organic, locally grown and sourced foods. You can look for labels that clearly state: USDA Organic, Non-GMO Project Verified, American Grass-Fed Association Certified, or Marine Stewardship Council. Also avoid preservatives, stabilizers, or added sugars in any food products you buy.

Pinpointing ultra-processed foods

When you are taking GLP-RA medications, you eat less overall and feel full faster, so there is much less room for "empty calories." Ultra-processed foods take up valuable stomach space without providing the protein, fiber, vitamins, and minerals your body needs to stay healthy during weight loss. They can also worsen common GLP-related side effects, such as: nausea, bloating, and reflux because they are often high in fat, sugar, or salt and low in fiber.

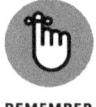

REMEMBER

Just follow this general rule: Any food with more than five ingredients is likely ultra-processed, particularly if you don't recognize those ingredients or you wouldn't use them in your own kitchen. These foods are typically nutrient-poor and are linked to additional health consequences such as blood sugar spikes, increased inflammation, poor gut health, and difficulty preserving lean muscle during weight loss. Examples include white sandwich bread with added sugars, flavored yogurts with thickeners and syrups, boxed rice or pasta mixes, and "protein" bars that are mostly sugar alcohols and additives. On GLP-RAs, choosing these foods makes it harder to meet your nutritional needs in a smaller volume of food, increasing the risk of fatigue, hair thinning, constipation, and nutrient deficiencies over time.

When scanning a food label, be cautious if you see several of the following ingredients, especially when they appear together or early in the list because they signal ultra-processed foods:

>> **Artificial flavors**

- Artificial colors (Red 40, Yellow 5, Blue 1)
- Sucralose, aspartame, acesulfame potassium (Ace-K)
- Carrageenan
- Polysorbate 80

>> **Preservatives**

- Sodium benzoate
- Potassium sorbate
- Calcium propionate
- BHA or BHT
- Sodium nitrite or nitrate (common in processed meats)

>> **Added sugars (often listed under multiple names)**

- High-fructose corn syrup
- Corn syrup or corn syrup solids
- Cane sugar, evaporated cane juice
- Dextrose, fructose, maltose
- Honey or agave syrup (still added sugar, despite the "natural" label)

>> **Refined starches and fillers**

- Enriched wheat flour
- Modified food starch
- Maltodextrin
- White rice flour
- Potato starch or tapioca starch (when used as fillers rather than whole foods)

>> **Highly processed oils**

- Soybean oil
- Corn oil
- Cottonseed oil
- Canola oil (especially when heavily refined or used in packaged foods)

TO EAT BREAD OR NOT EAT BREAD — THAT IS THE QUESTION

People who want to lose weight often wonder whether they can eat bread, and grocery store shelves are filled with ultra-processed bread, even though their labels make them sound like better choices. Examples of bread you should avoid include most packaged breads designed to be ultra-soft, shelf-stable, or slightly sweet. This commonly includes white sandwich bread made with enriched flour, added sugars, dough conditioners, and preservatives; "wheat" or "multigrain" breads where enriched flour is listed first despite healthy-sounding labels. Similarly, you should try to avoid low-calorie or "diet" breads that rely on modified starches, artificial fibers, and preservatives and shelf-stable hamburger buns, hot dog buns, and sub rolls. Shelf-stable breads use added sugars and refined oils to maintain texture and long shelf life and can disrupt the ability of your GLP–RA drug to work properly.

Defining a healthful dietary approach

A healthy approach to food ensures that your body receives the calories and nutrients it needs to function well, even when you are eating fewer calories for weight loss. To keep things running, you need two things:

>> **Calories** provide energy for essential processes such as breathing, circulation, digestion, movement, and temperature control.

>> **Nutrients** support muscle maintenance, hormone production, immune health, bone strength, and overall recovery.

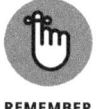

REMEMBER

When calorie intake decreases, nutrient needs remain the same, which makes food quality more important. This is especially important when using GLP–RA medications, because reduced appetite and smaller meals leave less room for foods that do not provide meaningful nutrition. Table 5-1 provides general calorie intake ranges based on different dietary goals to help you fuel your body while supporting safe and effective weight loss.

TABLE 5-1

Calorie Intake per Dietary Goal

Dietary Goal	Suggested Daily Calorie Intake
Weight loss (women)	1,200–1,500 calories/day
Weight loss (men)	1,500–1,800 calories/day
Weight maintenance	1,800–2,200 calories/day
Active lifestyle maintenance	2,200 calories/day

A well-balanced diet requires specific amounts of proteins, fats, and carbs depending on your activity level. Physical activity increases your body's demand for energy, muscle repair, and recovery, which directly affects how much of each macronutrient you need. People who are more active typically need more carbohydrates to fuel movement and workouts, as well as more protein to support muscle maintenance and repair. Those with lower activity levels may need fewer carbohydrates but still require adequate protein and healthy fats to preserve muscle, support hormones, and maintain overall health. Adjusting macronutrients to match activity level helps prevent fatigue, muscle loss, and poor recovery, especially when eating fewer calories for weight loss. Table 5-2 shows you how to balance all these nutrients based on your activity level. All nutrient amounts reflect the number of grams you should aim for per day per kilogram of your target body weight.

TABLE 5-2   ## Nutritional Intake per Activity Level

Activity Level	Protein (g/lb/day) (g/kg/day)	Fat (g/lb/day) (g/kg/day)	Carbs (g/lb/day) (g/kg/day)
Sedentary/low activity	0.55–0.64 (1.2–1.4)	0.36–0.45 (0.8–1.0)	1.14–1.36 (2.5–3.0)
Moderate activity	0.64–0.73 (1.4–1.6)	0.45–0.55 (1.0–1.2)	1.36–1.82 (3.0–4.0)
High activity	0.73–1.00 (1.6–2.2)	0.55–0.68 (1.2–1.5)	1.82–2.73 (4.0–6.0)

WARNING

While fiber is not a macronutrient, it remains an important part of a healthy diet. Most people do not get enough fiber, and GLP-RA medications can slow digestion, making adequate fiber intake especially helpful for regularity and reducing gastrointestinal side effects.

FIGURING MACRONUTRIENT GOALS

Macronutrient goals are typically calculated with guidance from a healthcare professional, such as a physician or registered dietitian, and are based on your body weight and activity level. Protein, fat, and carbohydrate needs are estimated using grams per kilogram of body weight per day, which are then converted to grams per day for practical use. This approach helps ensure you are getting enough energy and nutrients while eating fewer calories for weight loss. The ranges allow flexibility and can be adjusted based on physical activity, weight-loss rate, and how your body responds over time.

(continued)

(continued)

For example, a 130-pound person (about 59 kilograms) with a goal of losing about one to two pounds per week may have the following daily macronutrient targets:

- **Protein:** about 88 to 95 grams per day (based on 1.5 to 1.6 g/kg/day)

- **Fat:** about 65 to 71 grams per day (based on 1.1 to 1.2 g/kg/day)

- **Carbohydrates:** about 175 to 235 grams per day (based on 3.0 to 4.0 g/kg/day)

Creating Balanced, Satisfying Meals

TIP

Being on a GLP-RA medication essentially takes your appetite offline. And this situation affords you the opportunity to be very intentional about the foods you eat to ensure a nutrient rich diet.

Including important nutrients

To create a diet that includes appropriate calories and nutrients — but one that also gives you options — you can choose items from Table 5-3 and feel confident that you're meeting your nutritional needs (see the section earlier in this chapter, "Defining a healthful dietary approach" for more on your nutritional needs). We characterize the table as a GLP-RA choose-your-own-meal chart that offers you pre-selected, nutrient-dense foods. All you need to do is pick one selection from each column to create a balanced, high-protein, high-fiber meal.

TABLE 5-3   **GLP-RA Choose-Your-Own-Meal**

Protein (20–30g)	Vegetables (non-starchy, ~2g fiber/cup)	Fiber-Rich Carbs / Fat Add-Ins (4–8g fiber)
2 whole eggs + 2 egg whites (~22g protein)	Spinach	½ cup cooked sweet potato (~4g fiber, ~15g carb)
¾ cup Greek yogurt, plain (~17g protein)	Kale	¼ cup cooked lentils (~4g fiber, ~10g carb, +5g protein)
½ cup low-fat cottage cheese (~14g protein)	Romaine or butter lettuce	¼ cup quinoa, cooked (~2g fiber, ~10g carb, +6g protein)
1 can tuna in water (~20–25g protein)	Bok choy	1 tbsp chia seeds (~5g fiber, +2g protein)

Protein (20–30g)	Vegetables (non-starchy, ~2g fiber/cup)	Fiber-Rich Carbs / Fat Add-Ins (4–8g fiber)
4 oz grilled salmon (~24g protein)	Zucchini	1 tbsp ground flaxseed (~2g fiber, +1.5g protein)
4 oz grilled chicken breast (~26g protein)	Bell peppers	½ avocado (~5g fiber, healthy fat)
½ block tofu (~20g protein)	Cucumber	½ cup berries (~3–4g fiber, low sugar)
½ block tempeh (~17g protein)	Broccoli or cauliflower	1 slice spelt sourdough bread (~2g fiber, ~15g carb)
1 scoop protein powder* (~20–25g protein)	Green beans	1 tbsp pumpkin seeds (~2g fiber, +3g protein, healthy fat)

Mix in almond milk or water

Adding on the flavor

Of course, flavor helps enhance how satisfied you are with your food, and these items both add flavor and have other benefits. Be sure you stock your pantry with the following:

>> **Pantry staples:** Olive oil, salt, and pepper are everyday essentials you will use to flavor vegetables, lean proteins, and whole grains. Drizzle olive oil over roasted vegetables, grilled chicken, or fish, and use salt and pepper to season eggs, beans, soups, or sautéed greens. Olive oil also provides healthy fats that help with fullness and nutrient absorption.

>> **Lemon:** Nutritious and flavorful, lemon brightens dishes without adding calories. Use fresh lemon juice on fish, chicken, roasted vegetables, salads, or lentils to enhance flavor and reduce the need for heavy sauces. When cooking in cast iron, lemon also helps leach small amounts of iron from the pan into your food, which can help you meet a significant portion of your daily iron needs.

>> **Cinnamon:** This versatile spice adds natural sweetness and may help support more stable blood sugar levels. Sprinkle cinnamon on oatmeal, yogurt, cottage cheese, or fruit, or stir it into smoothies or warm beverages. It is especially useful for flavoring foods that might otherwise rely on added sugars.

>> **Turmeric:** With natural anti-inflammatory properties, turmeric adds warm, earthy flavor to meals. Use it in soups, stews, scrambled eggs, rice, lentils, roasted vegetables, or seasoning blends for chicken and fish. Pairing turmeric with a small amount of fat and black pepper helps improve its absorption.

>> **Saffron:** With mild anti-depressive properties, saffron has a mild, aromatic flavor and has been associated with mood-supporting properties. Use a small pinch in rice dishes, seafood, soups, or broths to add depth and richness without extra calories. A little goes a long way, making it a simple way to elevate basic meals.

Getting inspired by delicious ideas

Using Table 5-3 (see the section earlier in this chapter, "Including important nutrients"), you can mix and match proteins, vegetables, and fiber-rich add-ins to create satisfying meals throughout the day. When you put together meals, aim for the following each time to help you stay full, meet your nutrition needs, and keep calories in a reasonable range while on GLP-RA medications:

>> One protein (20 to 30mg)

>> One to two veggies

>> One fiber-rich carb or fat add-in (8 to 10g)

>> Total calories of 350 to 500

TIP

Cook in olive oil and season lightly with salt and pepper to taste.

These combinations not only meet your nutritional needs throughout the day, but they are also satisfying and delicious:

>> **Breakfast:**
  - Eggs with sweet potato hash
  - Greek yogurt with berries and chia seeds
  - Cottage cheese with cinnamon and berries
  - Protein shake mixed with almond milk and ground flaxseed

>> **Lunch:**
  - Tuna over romaine or butter lettuce with avocado
  - Grilled chicken with bell peppers and quinoa
  - Tofu with bok choy and lentils
  - Tempeh with cucumber, greens, and pumpkin seeds

» **Snack:**

- Greek yogurt with cinnamon and chia seeds
- Cottage cheese with berries
- Protein shake with almond milk
- Half an avocado with a slice of sourdough

» **Dinner:**

- Grilled salmon with zucchini and quinoa
- Chicken breast with broccoli or cauliflower and sweet potato
- Tofu stir-fry with green beans and lentils
- Tempeh with roasted vegetables and pumpkin seeds

THINKING HOLISTICALLY ABOUT HEALTH

Eating well is not just about what you put on your plate, but also about how food is prepared, stored, and handled. Everyday kitchen choices can affect your exposure to chemicals, plastics, and additives that may influence long-term health. These small changes support overall health by reducing unnecessary exposures while you focus on nourishing your body and support a cleaner eating environment:

- Use wooden or titanium cutting boards instead of plastic to help reduce microplastic particles that may shed into food during chopping.

- Store leftovers in glass containers rather than plastic to help limit chemical leaching, especially when food is warm or acidic.

- Cook using stainless steel, cast iron, or ceramic cookware instead of nonstick pans that may release chemicals when scratched or overheated.

- Avoid reheating food in plastic containers, as heat increases the transfer of chemicals into food.

- Wash fruits and vegetables thoroughly, or choosing organic options for produce with edible skins, can reduce pesticide residue.

Bottom line: Together, these practices complement a nutrient-dense diet and reinforce a holistic approach to health that supports well-being during weight loss and beyond.

Incorporating Physical Activity

Getting some physical activity in may sound daunting, but it's essential to your overall health and well-being. By the time you are 40, you begin losing 7 to 8 percent of your muscle per year, which is accelerated in women during perimenopause and menopause. In addition to combatting natural loss of muscle, GLP-RAs can hasten this process even more when you're cutting calories and not supplementing with protein. But protein supplementation only gets you so far — you need to turn that protein into muscle with strength training. In addition, general physical activity from walking not only helps with weight loss, but it can also improve digestion.

The goal here is to move more, sit less, and build muscle, but that doesn't mean hitting the gym for hours each day. In this section,

Getting yourself in motion with cardio

Cardiovascular activity helps your heart, lungs, and muscles work more efficiently and supports weight loss by increasing daily energy use. It also plays a key role in maintaining weight loss by helping prevent metabolic slowdown over time. Cardio does not have to mean running or intense workouts. Walking, cycling, swimming, rowing, or even dancing all count and can be adjusted to your fitness level and schedule. When paired with GLP-RA medications, regular cardio helps improve stamina, supports blood sugar control, and enhances overall well-being. Some of the more cardio-specific benefits on your body's well-being include:

>> **Lowers blood pressure:** Cardiovascular exercise improves blood vessel flexibility and reduces vascular resistance, allowing blood to flow more easily and decreasing the pressure exerted on artery walls.

>> **Improves sleep quality:** Regular cardio helps regulate circadian rhythms and increases adenosine buildup in the brain, which promotes deeper, more restorative sleep.

>> **Helps to control blood sugar:** Cardio increases glucose uptake by muscles and improves insulin sensitivity, allowing blood sugar to be used more efficiently for energy.

>> **Boosts mood and energy:** Aerobic activity stimulates the release of endorphins and neurotransmitters such as serotonin and dopamine, which enhance mood while improving oxygen delivery to tissues.

>> **Manages weight:** Cardiovascular exercise increases total daily energy expenditure and helps preserve metabolic rate during weight loss.

>> **Lowers your risk of chronic disease:** Regular cardio reduces inflammation, improves cholesterol profiles, enhances insulin sensitivity, and supports cardiovascular function, lowering the risk of conditions such as heart disease, type 2 diabetes, and stroke.

You might be imagining images of people sweating all over fancy cardio machines or getting up at the crack of dawn for a marathon-level run, but you shouldn't overthink or overdo cardio. Follow these tips to get yourself in motion and build this healthy habit into your lifestyle:

>> **Start small and simple.** The most sustainable way to begin cardio is to do a small amount of simple exercise each day. No need to get fancy gear or equipment. Go for fifteen-to-twenty-minute walks after meals. Then work your way up to about thirty to sixty minutes a day for five days a week. Starting with manageable, realistic movement helps your body adapt safely, reduces the risk of injury or burnout, and builds confidence over time. Small amounts of activity also work well with GLP-RA medications, which can temporarily affect energy levels, hydration, and tolerance for exertion.

>> **Break it up into chunks.** You don't have to carve out an hour of your day to get your cardio in. Just incorporate it into your everyday routine by finding small pockets of time to do a little bit. For example, stand up and stretch for two to three minutes every hour. Walk while talking on the phone. Walk around the parking lot or playing field where your kids are practicing. The steps will add up throughout the day.

>> **Track your steps to stay consistent.** Step tracking is one of the easiest ways to stay active throughout the day, and you can easily just use an app on your phone or a fitness tracker. Studies show that simply aiming to move more helps reduce body fat and improve blood sugar levels. Figure out your starting point. If you average 3,000 steps per day, aim for 4,000 next week, and then build up to 8,000 to 10,000 steps per day over time.

>> **Choose an activity that you enjoy.** You are more likely to stick with something if you enjoy doing it and it fits into your daily life.

TIP

We've created a sample cardio plan to show you how simple it can be. Feel free to swap workout types and activities for ones you enjoy doing or that fit into your current schedule:

>> **Monday:** Brisk walk for thirty minutes

>> **Tuesday:** Dance workout for twenty minutes

>> **Wednesday:** Rest or light stretching

>> **Thursday:** Bike ride or swim for thirty to forty-five minutes

>> **Friday:** Walk with a friend for thirty minutes

>> **Saturday:** Yard work or hike for forty-five to sixty minutes

>> **Sunday:** Rest

Building muscle with strength training

Strength training is an essential part of healthy aging and becomes even more important during weight loss. When you lose weight without strength training, your body does not just lose fat, it also loses valuable muscle mass. Loss of muscle can slow your metabolism, reduce strength, and make it harder to maintain weight loss over time. Building and preserving muscle helps your body burn calories more efficiently, supports balance and mobility, and protects against injury. Strength training also improves bone health and physical function, helping you stay strong, independent, and resilient as you age. Building muscle will help you:

>> **Burn fat:** Strength training helps build and preserve muscle, which increases your resting metabolic rate so your body burns more calories throughout the day, even when you are not exercising. This makes fat loss more efficient and helps prevent weight regain.

>> **Increase energy:** Regular strength training improves muscle efficiency and circulation, which can reduce fatigue and help you feel more energized during daily activities. Over time, having more muscle also means your body doesn't have to work as hard to do the same tasks.

>> **Reduce fall risk:** Strength training improves muscle strength, balance, and coordination, especially in the legs and core, which are critical for stability. Stronger muscles help you recover more quickly from slips or uneven surfaces, lowering the risk of falls and injuries.

>> **Make everyday tasks easier:** Building strength makes common activities like carrying groceries, climbing stairs, getting up from a chair, or lifting children feel easier and less tiring. This improved function supports independence and quality of life as you age.

If you think lifting weights, even using just your own body weight, is only for athletes or body builders, think again. Strength training is for everyone, and you don't have to build massive muscles to reap the benefits. If you follow these tips, you can make it sustainable, enjoyable, and beneficial for your weight-loss journey:

>> **Start with just your body weight.** Examples include chair squats, wall push-ups, step-ups on stairs, glute bridges, or standing calf raises while holding onto a counter for balance. These movements build foundational strength and confidence while reducing the risk of injury as your body adapts.

>> **Do just a few exercises per day at the beginning.** Starting with a small number of exercises helps prevent soreness and makes the habit easier to maintain. For example, you might choose two to three movements such as squats, push-ups, and planks one day, then lunges, rows with resistance bands, and bridges on another day. Keeping sessions short and focused allows strength to build gradually and sustainably over time.

>> **Break your workout up into chunks.** You can break your exercises up just like you would cardio instead of doing them all at once. When you're taking a break from work, get in a few sets of squats. Or before you sit down to watch your favorite show, do another set of exercises. You'll be surprised at how quickly and easily you can work these in throughout the day.

>> **Perform exercises, at first, that work major muscle groups.** Strength training can be overwhelming when you look at the lists of exercises you could perform. So start with ones that work major groups of muscles, like simple squats and shoulder press, to get the most out of your efforts. Then as you get stronger and motivated to increase what you're doing, you can fine-tune your workouts with other exercises.

>> **Maintain proper form to avoid injury.** If you aren't using a personal training or have access to a gym where they show you the ropes, just look online for videos of specific exercises so you can do them properly and not injure yourself.

>> **Increase weight gradually.** As your muscles adapt and exercises begin to feel easier, slowly increasing resistance helps you continue to build strength without overloading your joints or risking injury. A general recommendation during weight loss is to increase weight by about 5 to 10 percent at a time, only after you can complete all repetitions with good form and without excessive fatigue.

For example, if you start by lifting 20 pounds, a safe and realistic goal would be to gradually work up to 60 pounds over about 16 to 24 weeks, increasing the weight in small steps only after the exercise feels comfortable and your form remains strong.

This gradual progression supports muscle preservation and growth while allowing your body to recover appropriately, which is especially important when you are eating fewer calories. If weights are not available, you can also increase difficulty by adding repetitions, slowing the movement, or progressing from body-weight exercises to resistance bands before moving to heavier loads.

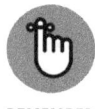

REMEMBER

If you already work out, maintain your current program for the first four weeks of being on a GLP-RA before trying to increase weight or reps. You may have less energy due to reduced caloric intake, so it's important not to over-stress your body.

TIP

You can use this simple circuit workout two to three times per week. Start with your body weight, then add small weight (five- or ten-pound dumbbells) as you get stronger. To complete a circuit, do the exercises in order but rest thirty to sixty seconds between exercises. It should feel challenging by the last few reps, but not painful. Remember that form matters more than speed. As you get stronger, increase reps first, then weights. For this circuit, complete two or three rounds of the following:

» 15 squats (pretend you're sitting on a chair)

» 15 bicep curls (use soup cans or light weights)

» 15 standing shoulder presses

» 10 to 15 modified push-ups (from knees, counter, or wall)

» 30-second plank (can be on knees)

TRAINING YOUR BODY THE RIGHT WAY

Weight loss ultimately depends on the balance between calories taken in and calories used or "burned." Each type of the following exercises offer unique benefits, and combining them leads to the best results for fat loss, muscle preservation, and overall health:

- **Cardio exercise,** such as walking, cycling, or swimming, steadily increases calorie use while improving heart and lung health.

- **Strength training** burns fewer calories during the workout itself but builds muscle that increases resting metabolism and supports long-term weight maintenance.

- **Circuit training** combines strength and cardio by moving quickly between exercises, which raises your heart rate while also building muscle and improving efficiency.

- **High-intensity interval training (HIIT)** alternates short bursts of intense effort with recovery periods and has been shown to improve cardiovascular fitness and insulin sensitivity in less time.

The most effective and widely recommended approach to weight loss is to combine cardio and strength training, rather than choosing just one type of exercise. National guidelines, including those from the CDC and American College of Sports Medicine, recommend at least 150 minutes of moderate-intensity cardio per week plus two or more days of strength training, as this combination best supports fat loss, muscle preservation, metabolic health, and long-term weight maintenance.

Considering Supplements While Taking GLP-RAs

Key nutrient deficiencies may emerge while on GLP-RAs, especially if your diet is not optimized with nutrient-dense foods (see the section earlier in this chapter, "Rethinking Nutrition and Diet," for more on the nutrients you need). Below is a list of common nutrient deficiencies you may experience while on GLP-RAs, and we list symptoms to watch for as well as what sources can help you ensure you get enough of these vital nutrients:

>> **Vitamin B12:** Symptoms of vitamin B12 deficiency include fatigue, brain fog, and tingling, but eggs, meat, dairy, and fortified foods are good sources of this nutrient.

>> **Iron:** Symptoms of an iron deficiency include weakness and sensitivity to cold, but red meat, spinach, and legumes are good sources of iron.

>> **Vitamin D:** Symptoms of vitamin D deficiency include low mood and bone pain, but sunlight and fatty fish are good sources of vitamin D.

>> **Magnesium:** Symptoms of magnesium deficiency include cramps, insomnia, and headaches, but leafy greens, nuts, and dark chocolate are good sources of magnesium.

>> **Zinc:** Symptoms of a zinc deficiency include poor healing and taste changes, but shellfish, seeds, and legumes are good sources of zinc.

REMEMBER

It may not be possible to consume enough to keep up with all of these nutrients, so you may need to consider the following supplements. Talk to your doctor about your specific needs for:

>> **Collagen and a hair multivitamin:** In a calorie-restricted state, your body may prioritize essential functions over skin and hair health, which can lead to hair thinning or changes in skin quality. Collagen and hair-focused multivitamins may help support hair strength, skin elasticity, and nail health during weight loss.

- **A multivitamin with folate, B12, magnesium, iron, vitamin K2, and vitamin D:** When calorie intake is reduced, it can be difficult to consistently meet micronutrient needs through food alone. A comprehensive multivitamin may help prevent deficiencies that can affect energy levels, bone health, red blood cell production, and overall well-being. See CH3 for more information.

- **Magnesium glycinate:** Women, specifically, may benefit from magnesium glycinate, particularly around ovulation when magnesium stores can be lower and sleep may be disrupted. This form of magnesium is well absorbed and may help support sleep quality, muscle relaxation, and stress regulation.

- **B-complex vitamin:** B vitamins play a key role in energy metabolism and nervous system function and may help reduce fatigue during periods of increased physical activity or calorie restriction. They can be especially helpful when starting a new exercise routine.

TIP

Monitor your ferritin (marker of iron stores), B12, basic metabolic panel, folate, and vitamin D levels every three to six months. Chapter 6 can tell you more details on what you need to monitor with your doctor and why.

Gut health is key for optimizing your mood, immune system, and inflammation. Your gut is a central hub where 80 percent of your immune system cells are produced and where over 90 percent of your serotonin, your feel-good hormone, is produced. GLP-RAs can lead to slowed digestion due to delayed gastric emptying and can also trigger indigestion and constipation, so a healthy gut microbiome is key. To keep your get in check, consider a combination of pre-, pro-, and postbiotics from your food to support your gut:

- **Prebiotics:** This is the food the good bacteria in our gut need to survive. They are non-digestible fibers found in garlic, onions, leeks, asparagus, oats, and bananas. They can also help to improve insulin sensitivity.

- **Probiotics:** This is the good bacteria itself, such as lactobacillus and acidophilus which can be found in certain fermented foods, such as kefir and yogurt.

- **Postbiotics:** These are the byproducts that good bacteria produce to support the gut and digestive lining, and they are also found in fermented foods. Butyrate is one of those byproducts, which supports the lining of the colon, and research suggests it can help with leaky gut.

TECHNICAL
STUFF

Leaky gut is increased intestinal permeability, meaning that the cells lining the gut are unhealthy, so toxins, bacteria, and food byproducts can leak out into the blood stream triggering inflammation and even autoimmune issues.

TAKING NATURAL SUPPLEMENTS TO SUPPORT WEIGHT LOSS

Many people look to natural supplements when weight-loss medications are not an option, are not well tolerated, or do not provide the full results they hoped for. Others use supplements as an addition to GLP-RA therapy to support fullness, blood sugar control, gut health, or metabolic function. It is important to understand that supplements *do not* replace GLP-RAs, surgery, or structured lifestyle programs. Their effects are modest and work best when combined with healthy eating, regular movement, and behavior change. Examples include fiber supplements to improve fullness and appetite control, green tea extract to slightly increase fat oxidation, probiotics to support gut health and reduce visceral fat, berberine to improve insulin sensitivity, and omega-rich dietary patterns that support metabolic health.

Before taking any of these supplements, discuss them with your doctor to make sure they are safe, appropriate, and compatible with your medications and weight-loss plan. Popular natural supplements include:

- **Green tea** contains a powerful antioxidant called EGCG (epigallocatechin gallate), which has been shown to boost fat oxidation and improve insulin sensitivity. It may also increase energy expenditure and reduce body fat, especially in the abdominal area. Just choose decaffeinated if you're sensitive to caffeine and avoid high doses because of the potential for liver toxicity.

- **Berberine** is a plant compound that has been suggested to support weight loss, however randomized clinical trials are lacking and research to date has had a high degree of bias. It may reduce fasting glucose and improve insulin sensitivity and help prevent weight regain during maintenance phases. However, it may interact with medications, so do not combine with GLP-RAs without supervision.

- **Fiber supplements (like psyllium husk or glucomannan)** slow digestion, improve satiety, and supports gut health — all of which can amplify the appetite-suppressing effects of GLP-RAs.

- **Cinnamon** has been studied for its potential to improve blood sugar levels and insulin sensitivity. It may reduce fasting glucose and enhance insulin response.

- **Probiotics** may support weight management by improving gut bacteria balance, reducing inflammation, and slightly improving how the body processes fat and sugar. Certain strains, such as *Lactobacillus gasseri* SBT2055, have been shown to produce small reductions in body weight, body mass index, waist size, and visceral fat over about twelve weeks. Other strains, including *Lactobacillus plantarum*

(continued)

(continued)

KY1032, have shown similar modest benefits compared with placebo. Overall weight loss is usually small, often around one to three kilograms, so probiotics should be viewed as a supportive add-on rather than a primary weight-loss tool. Benefits are strain-specific, so results may vary, and probiotics work best when combined with healthy eating, regular movement, and other proven strategies.

Natural supplements can offer small, supportive benefits for weight management, but they are not a replacement for medications, procedures, or lifestyle changes. When used thoughtfully and under medical guidance, they may help reinforce fullness, metabolic health, or weight maintenance alongside a comprehensive plan. To learn more about evidence-based alternatives and adjuncts to weight-loss medications, read on to Chapter 13 for a deeper discussion.

Chapter **6**

Monitoring and Maintaining Success with Tests and Tech

Technology has become a powerful partner in your weight-loss journey. Especially when taking GLP RA medications, technology can offer you safe enhancement strategies that make tracking, planning, and staying motivated for weight loss easier than ever. This chapter will provide a walkthrough of various consumer-based websites and online programs you may find helpful.

These technology adjuncts provide education and community support for weight loss, deliver real-time feedback on your activity, sleep, and health trends in the form of wearables, and even analyze your calorie intake using artificial intelligence (AI). Artificial intelligence adds the newest technology layer to your journey by personalizing calorie tracking, suggesting healthier choices, and predicting when you might need extra support.

REMEMBER

However, while these technologies are helpful, they are simply tools for you to use. You must also commit to a safety monitoring program with regular blood-lab follow up with your medical team to protect your health and sustain your results.

Using Apps and Wearables

First and foremost, a successful weight-loss journey requires vigilant tracking. Tracking your habits can be one of the most powerful things you do. Technology, apps, and wearables can help you monitor your food, movement, sleep, and medication to enhance your awareness. That awareness helps you make better choices, especially when motivation runs low.

Smart device mobile apps

Several mobile apps can help you remember to take your medications, including Medisafe, MyTherapy, and Dosecast. Research on Medisafe has shown improved self-reported adherence in patients with chronic conditions, with one randomized study noting a 7 percent increase in medication-taking behavior compared to controls. Whether you're taking your GLP-RA once a day or once a week, these apps can help you maintain pique awareness to take your medicine at the right time, every time. MyTherapy has also demonstrated high user satisfaction and better adherence in patients with multiple medications in observational studies, while Dosecast is widely used but lacks large-scale published trials.

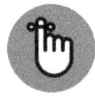

REMEMBER

You don't need to be perfect, but you do need to be consistent, and these apps can help make that happen when you build them into your regular routine.

TIP

These apps are helpful because they make it easier to stick to your goals, especially when life gets busy. When you incorporate these tools to your weight-loss routine, it can feel like adding a new team member to your weight-loss journey. The task of "remembering" to take your medicines, complete your exercise, or maintain your diet is no longer your responsibility alone.

Research shows that smartphone apps can be effective tools in supporting weight loss, especially when they include features like self-monitoring, goal setting, reminders, and feedback. A meta-analysis by Islam et al. (2020) found that mobile health (mHealth) interventions using smartphone apps led to significant reductions in body weight, with an average weight loss of 2.68 kg (nearly 6 pounds) compared to control groups. Apps that incorporated daily self-monitoring of diet and physical activity showed the greatest benefit.

Another study by Carter et al. (2013) demonstrated that users who tracked their food intake using mobile apps lost more weight than those using paper diaries or websites. These tools improve accountability, reinforce healthy behaviors, and help users detect early patterns that may lead to setbacks. While not a substitute for medical care, Apps can play a strong supportive role in your long-term weight management especially when your build them into your daily routine and use these tools consistently.

Online programs

Even with the best care team, you might need more, and you don't need to do this alone. Online weight-loss programs can provide structure, education, and community support that add more dimension and success to your weight-loss journey.

Online weight-loss programs and calorie counters can offer structure, education, and a sense of community, making it easier for you to stay on track. Free options like MyFitnessPal (basic version) and Lose It! (basic version) provide calorie tracking, goal setting, and integration with wearables. Similarly, you have access to paid programs like Noom, Weight Watchers (WW), and MyFitnessPal Premium which add coaching, personalized plans, and behavioral tools to their platforms. Research shows that programs combining calorie tracking, group support, and behavior-change strategies tend to produce the best results. Choosing between free and paid options depends on your need for guidance, accountability, and extra features to maintain motivation over time.

Table 6-1 summarizes the three most commonly used online and community programs available to you for weight loss, using results obtained from open-access, online sources, not published research data.

TABLE 6-1   ## What to Expect from Popular Online Programs

Program	Short-Term Effectiveness	Long-Term Success
Weight Watchers (points-based behavioral program)	Participants lose 5 to 10 percent of weight within 6 to 12 months	Sustained weight loss seen at two years
Noom (behavior-focused)	5 to 7 percent average loss in six months	Early data suggest durable habit change
Nutrisystem (less structured long-term)	Quick results	Weight regain common after stopping program

Wearable technologies

Wearables like the Apple Watch, Fitbit, Garmin, and WHOOP can do much more than count your steps. You can unlock powerful insights with just a little know-how.

Many of these types of devices have been shown to support weight loss by promoting self-monitoring, increasing daily activity, and providing real-time feedback. A systematic review and meta-analysis by Cheatham and team in 2018 found that activity trackers were associated with significant increases in physical activity and modest but meaningful weight loss. Similarly, a large randomized controlled trial in 2016 reported that wearables alone may not outperform traditional behavioral programs. The study did show that wearable technologies can enhance motivation and adherence when integrated into a structured weight-loss plan. This may present an opportunity for you to pair multiple platforms together like community-based programs, such as Weight Watchers, with wearables and your weight-loss medicines.

REMEMBER

The continuous data from wearables like steps, heart rate, and sleep help you to track your weight-loss medicines and progress, adjust goals, and identify patterns that could hinder your success. When paired with coaching or app-based feedback, wearables become powerful tools for sustaining your lifestyle changes that support your long-term weight control.

Here are the main metrics that these devices can capture that you should look for and track:

>> **Sleep duration:** Poor sleep increases hunger hormones and reduces insulin sensitivity.

>> **Sleep quality:** Detect sleep disorders like apnea.

>> **Heart rate variability:** A marker of stress and recovery, low HRV is linked to poorer outcomes.

>> **Active minutes:** Track how much you're really moving, not just your steps.

>> **Blood oxygen levels:** You might discover undiagnosed sleep apnea or nighttime breathing problems.

TIP

Many newer devices can even screen for Obstructive Sleep Apnea (OSA). If your wearable shows low oxygen levels at night, or if you feel tired even after a full night's sleep, it might be time to talk to your doctor. Your doctor may need to order a *polysomnography* (a sleep study). A sleep study is a test that monitors your breathing, heart rate, and oxygen while you sleep. If OSA is diagnosed, you may be prescribed a Continuous Positive Airway Pressure (CPAP) machine. The CPAP machine can help you breathe better at night, which leads you to improved energy, weight loss, and focus.

Wearable devices can be helpful tools during weight loss, not because they "burn calories for you," but because they provide feedback that supports awareness, consistency, and habit formation. No single device is best for everyone. The most useful option depends on what you want to track and how much data you find helpful rather than overwhelming. Below is a simple overview of popular wearables and how they may support people using GLP–RA medications:

>> **Apple Watch:** If you want comprehensive health tracking, this device has strong app integration and provides motivational prompts. For people on GLP-RAs, this can support daily step goals, gentle device-automated activity reminders, and awareness of trends without requiring advanced setup. It works best for users who already rely heavily on their phone and prefer simple, automated feedback. This device does support customer-directed feedback as well in the form of user created reminders.

>> **Fitbit:** The most practical in terms of cost, this device still gives you a lot of support when managing your weight loss. Fitbit is a straightforward option for people who mainly want step counts, activity tracking, and sleep data without complexity. Setup is simple, and the interface is easy to understand, making it a good choice for those focused on building consistency rather than analyzing performance. For GLP-RA users, Fitbit can help reinforce daily movement goals and track sleep patterns that may change with weight loss. It pairs well with basic lifestyle goals and does not require frequent interaction to be effective. Different from the Apple Watch, Fitbit has less potential for specific, user-directed goal setting and reminders beyond steps and activity level.

>> **Garmin:** Another option for comprehensive health tracking, the Garmin line works with both Apple and Android devices. Specifically, you could consider the Garmin Forerunner. Garmin devices are highly functional and durable, including for water-based activities such as swimming and rowing. They offer detailed activity tracking, heart-rate data, and performance metrics while still allowing basic step and movement goals. Many athletes and highly active individuals prefer Garmin for its reliability and flexibility, but it also works well for beginners who want accurate movement tracking. Garmin devices integrate easily with apps like Strava, which can add motivation through social support and progress tracking.

>> **Oura Ring:** If you're wanting something more discreet, this device is your best fit. The Oura Ring is designed to focus primarily on sleep, recovery, and readiness rather than step counts or workouts. It provides insight into sleep quality, resting heart rate, and recovery trends, which can be useful for people on GLP-RAs who experience fatigue or changes in sleep patterns. This device may be best for those who prefer minimal interaction and want health insights without wearing a watch. The ring can detect different activity types beyond traditional cycling or strength workouts including skiing and horse-back riding.

TIP

Wearables work best not as passive trackers, but as daily feedback tools you respond to. Focus on just one or two simple metrics at a time, such as daily steps or active minutes, to avoid data overload and improve consistency. Use reminders or gentle prompts as cues to move, hydrate, or wind down for sleep, rather than as pressure to "hit perfect numbers." Most importantly, review your trends weekly and adjust habits gradually, since small, repeated changes lead to the best long–term results during GLP–RA–supported weight loss.

DO WEARABLES WORK?

Wearables used to be athlete-only tech reserved for marathoners, cyclists, and people who lived inside performance dashboards. But today, you see them everywhere. Smartwatches, rings, and sensor-equipped clothing promise to track everything from steps and heart rate to sleep quality and blood glucose trends. But do they actually help with weight loss?

The research is mixed: Wearables reliably measure activity, sleep, and other health markers, but their impact on long-term weight change depends on how people use the data. Here's what studies show about what wearables do well — and where their limits are:

- **Step-count wearables:** A 2019 study by Brickwood and team showed that people using step-count wearable devices increased their daily physical activity compared with those who did not use a device. Higher daily movement supports weight-loss efforts and is especially important for maintaining weight loss over time.

- **Fitbit:** A 2016 study by Jakicic and team showed that adding a Fitbit to a standard behavioral weight-loss program did not produce greater long-term weight loss compared with counseling alone. However, the device was effective for tracking physical activity, reinforcing its role as a habit-support tool rather than a stand-alone weight-loss solution.

- **Oura Ring:** A 2021 study by Altini and team showed that the Oura Ring measured total sleep time and sleep stages with accuracy similar to clinical sleep-monitoring methods. Because sleep quality influences appetite, energy, and weight regulation, reliable sleep tracking can help support healthier routines during weight loss.

- **Hexoskin:** A 2017 study by Montalvo and team showed that the Hexoskin wearable accurately measured heart rate and breathing when compared with laboratory-based testing. Accurate tracking of these signals can help users better understand exercise intensity and recovery, supporting safer and more effective physical activity.

- **Continuous glucose monitors (CGM):** A 2019 study by Riddell and team showed that using continuous glucose monitoring improved dietary awareness and food choices in athletes. Increased awareness of blood sugar responses may help some individuals make nutrition decisions that better support metabolic health and weight management.

- **Vital-sign monitoring patches:** A 2020 study by Weenk and team showed that wearable patch devices accurately tracked vital signs such as heart rate and breathing over time. These findings support the broader reliability of wearable technologies used to monitor health trends relevant to activity, recovery, and overall well-being.

The bottom line: Like any tool, how you use it matters most. You'll find the most success if you pair the data with intentional habits, such as planning meals based on CGM insights, using sleep scores to adjust bedtime routines, or setting step and heart-rate targets you check and act on.

Maximizing Results with Artificial Intelligence

Artificial intelligence (AI) works by using computer programs called algorithms to quickly analyze patterns in data and make smart predictions or suggestions. With respect to your weight-loss journey, AI can give personalized tips, meal plans, or activity goals to help you lose weight more effectively. These sections reveal just how AI can be a helpful tool for your goals.

Grasping how AI can help

AI has opened exciting new ways to track and manage your health. AI-powered apps can analyze meals from photos, calculate calories, and even recommend recipes that meet your goals. And AI is already integrated into websites like MyFitnessPal, Lumen, and Noom, which use AI to give you personalized feedback based on your habits. Some AI tools even connect to your wearable devices to monitor your sleep and activity.

AI can also help:

>> **Identify emotional eating patterns:** You likely don't realize how or why you're eating, but when AI offers you feedback, you can adjust and make positive changes to support your weight loss.

>> **Suggest healthier food swaps or portion sizes:** AI can take into account what you've consumed throughout the day and help you adjust to your unique needs.

>> **Predict when you're likely to slip:** This is key — AI can remind you before slip-ups happen! Remember, everyone slips up, but AI can help prevent it from being a setback to your weight-loss goals.

>> **Explain normal weight fluctuations:** Daily changes on the scale can be confusing and discouraging. AI can help explain when weight changes are likely due to hydration, sodium intake, digestion, or hormonal shifts rather than true fat gain, helping you stay focused on long-term progress.

>> **Encourage consistency with habits:** AI can prompt gentle reminders to drink water, move your body, eat regular meals, or prioritize sleep based on your daily patterns. These small nudges help reinforce healthy routines without feeling judgmental or overwhelming.

>> **Provide motivation and support during tough days:** When motivation dips, AI can offer reassurance, normalize setbacks, and help you reframe challenges. Feeling supported, even digitally, can make it easier to stay engaged and committed to your weight-loss journey.

WARNING

AI tools are meant to support habits, motivation, and self-awareness, not to replace medical care or provide medical advice. They should never discourage you from checking in with your healthcare team or seeking professional guidance for symptoms, side effects, or concerns during your weight-loss journey.

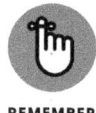

REMEMBER

AI can make mistakes. Any AI-created recommendations you receive which tell you to start, stop, or change your medicines should be discussed with your doctor, first.

Taking advantage of AI integration

TIP

AI is increasingly being used in weight-loss programs to help guide your day-to-day decisions and support healthy habits. When used appropriately, it can offer reminders, insights, and encouragement that make your weight-loss journey easier and more sustainable. AI-powered apps and platforms can analyze dietary patterns, activity levels, and even emotional triggers to create individualized recommendations in real time.

A systematic review by Elhussein et al. in 2023 concluded that AI-based tools, including chatbots and predictive models, significantly improved adherence to dietary and exercise goals. This means you can combine your medicines with help from AI to achieve measurable weight loss. Another randomized controlled trial using an AI virtual health coach (Lark) showed improved dietary behaviors and sustained weight reduction over twelve weeks in 2017.

REMEMBER

These technologies offer scalable and low-cost support, particularly when combined with wearables (see the earlier section, "Wearable technologies" for more) that feed your data continuously into the AI algorithms. While AI doesn't replace clinical care, it enhances self-management and accountability. These are some of your most critical weight-loss monitoring elements for long-term weight success.

Tracking food and calories with AI

You may realize that counting your own meal and snack calories is quite the time-consuming task. For some people, calorie counting takes a huge amount of commitment and mental effort, but it is a key task for a successful weight-loss journey. AI-powered calorie counting uses machine learning and image recognition to estimate the nutritional content of your meals using a meal photo or short description of the meal by text. These systems pull from large food databases, recipe datasets, and USDA nutrient information, and they learn to match food images with portion sizes and nutritional values.

Several weight-loss apps now use artificial intelligence to make tracking food easier and more accurate. For example, MyFitnessPal Premium uses barcode scanning, image recognition, and even natural language input to speed up logging. Lose It! Snap It allows you to simply take a photo of your meal, and AI suggests the food and portion size. Bite.ai works as a chatbot that can recognize foods from either pictures or written descriptions. CalorieMama estimates calories from meal photos using deep-learning models trained on millions of food images, while PlateMate combines AI with crowd-sourced verification to identify foods and portion sizes from uploaded photos.

AI calorie counting can be quite accurate for packaged foods (often within 5 to 10 percent of actual values) when barcode scanning is used, because it pulls directly from nutrition labels. For home-cooked or restaurant meals, accuracy is lower — typically 20 to 30 percent — due to variability in portion size and recipe ingredients, but AI's precision improves when users confirm or adjust entries. Here's a look at the AI tools that do this best:

>> **Bite.ai:** Bite.ai is free and focuses on simplicity and ease of use. It allows users to log meals through text or photos using an AI chatbot, reducing the burden of manual entry. However, it does not provide detailed nutrient breakdowns or long-term trend analysis.

>> **CalorieMama:** The free version allows users to log foods using photo recognition and track daily calorie intake. The upgraded version costs

about $29.99 per year and includes more detailed nutrition information, a larger food database, and improved accuracy for mixed meals. Paid features also help identify eating patterns over time.

>> **Cronometer:** The free version offers detailed calorie and micronutrient tracking, including many vitamins and minerals. The Gold version costs about $49.99 per year and adds advanced customization, long-term trend analysis, and flexible goal setting. It is especially useful for users focused on nutrient adequacy during calorie restriction.

>> **Lose It! (Snap It):** The free version lets you log meals, track calories, and use photo-based food logging with limited nutrient detail. The paid version costs about $39.99 per year and expands nutrient tracking, allows more personalized calorie and macronutrient targets, and offers progress reports and pattern insights. These features help support habit building and long-term consistency.

>> **MyFitnessPal:** The free version allows you to log foods, track calories, and view basic macronutrients like protein, carbohydrates, and fat. The premium version costs about $79.99 per year and adds more detailed nutrient tracking, including fiber, sodium, sugar, and selected vitamins and minerals, which can be especially helpful when eating fewer calories on GLP-RA medications. Premium also allows customizable macronutrient goals and provides insights and trend reports that help explain plateaus or weight fluctuations.

>> **PlateMate:** PlateMate uses a subscription-based pricing model, with costs varying by plan. Paid access provides a hybrid of AI analysis and crowd-sourced insight to estimate portion sizes and nutritional content, especially for restaurant meals. This can be helpful for users who prefer visual guidance rather than precise food weighing.

TIP

AI calorie counting works best when you pair it with quick user verification. While AI can dramatically speed up logging and reduce missed entries, human input is still important for high accuracy. Choose the level of tracking that matches your goals and tolerance for detail. Many people do well starting with a free version and upgrading only if they want deeper insight into nutrients and long-term trends.

TECHNICAL
STUFF

Even newer AI tools make tracking your meals as simple as snapping a photo. For example, systems like Im2Calories can recognize what's on your plate and estimate calories when linked to restaurant menus. Other tools use advanced deep-learning neural networks to figure out food type, ingredients, and calorie count all at once for better accuracy. Some even use creative AI models, called Generative Adversarial Networks (GANs), to guess portion sizes and calorie content from a single picture with surprising precision.

REMEMBER

Using AI for calorie counting is probably more accurate than asking your friends. Studies show that most people are way off when guessing calories from food photos. People are only correct about 20 percent of the time. On the other hand, AI can get much closer to the real number, making it a powerful helper for your weight-loss journey.

Using AI prompts effectively

AI works best when you think of it as a conversation rather than a single-use question-and-answer tool. The quality of what you get back depends largely on how you ask, the quality of information you give it, and how you follow up. Clear prompts help AI give more relevant, personalized, and useful guidance. By refining your questions over time, you will be able to generate better results. Instead of asking one broad question and stopping there, you can clarify, redirect, or ask for examples to get information that fits your needs.

Keep these tips in mind while chatting with AI:

>> **Be specific.** Asking AI, "Help me lose weight," will give you less satisfying results than, "Help me create a seven-day meal plan at 1,200 calories a day with nutrient-dense food." So be specific about what you're wanting to discover when you engage with AI.

>> **Add personal context.** AI can tailor recommendations to your weight, schedule, and dietary needs. The more AI knows about you, the better its ideas and feedback will be. For example, if you do not like kale but want to try quinoa, you can say that and get better meal ideas. If you have challenges with exercise, AI can help you work around them and suggest ways to stay active.

>> **Use prompts to create actionable steps.** You can get more than just information from AI. It can also synthesize what you've asked and what your goals are and give you steps to reach them. For example, if you tell AI what your schedule is like and explain that you want to increase your steps each week gradually until you hit 5,000, it can give you a plan to reach that goal while balancing the rest of your schedule and life events.

>> **Refine the answers.** Some people give up on AI because it doesn't give the perfect response the first time. So ask follow-up questions. If the response you're given isn't digestible or easily acted upon, then ask for adjustments, set parameters, ask for more details, and so on until you get the actionable, ready-to-use information you need.

>> **Use AI as a partner, not a decision-maker.** Get the most out of your AI experience by not relying on it to command your every move or decision. Instead, use it for collaboration. Ask for AI to offer considerations about a decision you're making, to list things you're not thinking of, and so on — don't simply hand over control.

Even if you've never used AI before, you can easily put together prompts so that you have robust conversations that offer you actionable information. Just follow these steps to create prompts that offer you tailored, practical guidance:

1. **Start with the outcome you want.** Tell AI the job you want it to do. It sounds obvious, but it's easy to overlook this step, especially if you're overwhelmed by information. So ask it to summarize your weekly activity data into bullet points or build a meal plan for someone with a lower appetite on GLP-1 medications.

2. **Add context.** You do not need to share your full medical history. You do need to share details that matter for your question. If you exercise regularly but have a busy day, you can ask for a workout that is split into short sessions. If you want a meal plan, you can share your weight, activity level, and weight-loss goal.

3. **List constraints.** Without offering some boundaries, you'll have to narrow the information yourself, which isn't efficient. Clear boundaries help you get useful answers faster. For example, if you cannot eat dairy, only want free apps, or need beginner friendly exercises. Save time and reduce confusion by telling AI.

4. **Ask for structure.** Structure makes information easier to use. You can ask for steps, short lists, or a plan broken into smaller parts. This helps you act on the information right away.

Taking Regular Laboratory Tests

You can't fix what you don't measure, and that includes your internal health. Routine lab testing isn't just about you checking boxes. This practice is a commitment to the gold-standard monitoring recommended for patients on weight-loss medications, especially GLP-RAs. The information gained helps you and your doctor make key decisions about your weight-loss journey to ensure the treatment plan is helping, not hurting, the rest of your body.

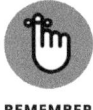

REMEMBER

Regular lab work helps you keep track of your health by monitoring for medication side effects, showing how your body is responding to weight loss, and catching potential problems. When you catch problems related to excess weight early, different diseases and potential complications like diabetes, nutrient deficiencies, or organ stress are often easier to manage.

Answering the who, what, and when for lab tests

To understand how your body is responding to treatment, you need to get lab tests done at different intervals while on your GLP–RA medication. Your doctor will compare these to the baseline levels tested before you began treatment. (Chapter 3 gives you more information about what screenings you need and why.)

Here are the tests you'll have done and when they need to be performed:

>> **A1C and fasting glucose:** These tests help assess blood sugar control and identify diabetes or prediabetes. Check at baseline before starting a GLP-RA, then repeat every three to six months to monitor response to treatment.

>> **Lipid panel:** This test evaluates cholesterol levels and overall cardiovascular risk, which often improve with weight loss. Check at baseline, then repeat annually while on GLP-RA therapy.

>> **Liver function tests (LFTs):** These screen for fatty liver disease, liver inflammation, or medication-related effects. Check at baseline, then repeat if symptoms arise or if there are clinical concerns.

>> **Kidney function (creatinine and estimated glomerular filtration rate):** These tests assess kidney health and hydration status, which is important because nausea or reduced intake on GLP-RAs can affect fluid balance. Check at baseline, then annually.

>> **TSH and free T4:** These tests evaluate thyroid function, which can affect metabolism, energy, and weight changes. Check at baseline, then repeat if symptoms such as fatigue, hair loss, or temperature intolerance develop.

>> **Vitamin B12:** This test monitors for deficiency, especially in people taking metformin or those with fatigue, numbness, or tingling. Check at baseline, then every one to two years or sooner if symptoms appear.

>> **25-Hydroxy vitamin D and calcium:** These tests help monitor bone health during weight loss, particularly in people at risk for deficiency. Check at baseline, then every six to twelve months if risk factors are present.

>> **Iron studies (ferritin, total iron-binding capacity, and iron):** These tests detect iron deficiency that may result from low intake or absorption during weight loss. Check at baseline, then repeat if fatigue, hair loss, or other symptoms develop.

TIP

Your doctor should be keeping tabs on these labs and making sure they are ordered and reviewed. But if you do not have insurance or do not connect regularly with a healthcare provider, you still have options. Companies like QuestDirect, Ulta Lab Tests, Everlywell, and Walk-In Lab offer direct-to-consumer blood testing without requiring a doctor's visit. These services can help you access important monitoring while on GLP-RA medications. This is also an opportunity to pair with telehealth and digital weight-loss consultation platforms, such as Hims. (See Chapter 3 for more information on these platforms.)

Responding to abnormal labs

When any of your labs are out of range, you should not panic. You can use this information as a signal to dig deeper and make adjustments where necessary. Lab results are best viewed as information, not a diagnosis, and they often signal an opportunity to make small, helpful adjustments. If you have a doctor, they will usually review abnormal results with you and recommend next steps, which may include repeat testing, lifestyle changes, or supplements. If you do not have insurance or a regular provider, you can use telehealth services or direct-to-consumer lab companies paired with medical consultation to help interpret results. The key message is this: Abnormal labs should guide a conversation with a healthcare professional, not prompt you to treat yourself without guidance.

Here's an idea of what to expect:

>> **If your A1C or fasting glucose is high:** This may mean you have diabetes or are very close to it. Your doctor may order additional blood tests to better understand how your body is making and using insulin or refer you to a diabetes specialist. They may also talk with you about nutrition, activity, and medication options to improve blood sugar control.

>> **If your cholesterol or triglycerides are high:** Your doctor may explain how these numbers affect your heart and blood vessel health and look at your overall cardiovascular risk. They may recommend changes in diet, physical activity, or medications and may want to repeat the labs after several months to see how they respond to weight loss and treatment.

>> **If your liver tests are elevated:** This can be a sign of fat buildup or inflammation in the liver, which is common with excess weight and insulin resistance. Your doctor may order imaging tests of the liver or refer you to a liver specialist to better understand what is going on. Weight loss often improves these numbers over time.

>> **If kidney function tests are abnormal:** This may suggest that your kidneys are under strain or not filtering as well as expected. Your doctor may repeat

the tests, review your hydration and medications, and decide whether a kidney specialist should be involved. Staying well hydrated is often emphasized.

» **If thyroid tests are abnormal:** Your doctor may repeat the tests or order additional blood work to look for autoimmune thyroid conditions. Thyroid problems can affect energy, metabolism, and weight, so your doctor may refer you to an endocrinologist for further evaluation.

» **If vitamin B12 levels are low:** Low B12 can contribute to fatigue, weakness, or nerve symptoms. Your doctor may recommend supplementation and follow-up testing to make sure levels improve, especially if you take medications that affect absorption.

» **If vitamin D or calcium levels are low:** Your doctor may discuss bone health and recommend lifestyle changes or supplements to support bone strength during weight loss. Follow-up testing is often used to make sure levels return to a healthy range.

» **If iron levels are low:** This can contribute to fatigue, shortness of breath, or hair thinning. Your doctor may look for reasons such as low intake or absorption and discuss dietary changes or supplementation, along with repeat testing. Read more in depth about the importance of iron in the later section, "Addressing iron deficiency anemia."

Addressing iron deficiency anemia

Iron deficiency anemia occurs when your body does not have enough iron to make healthy red blood cells, which are needed to carry oxygen throughout the body. This condition is more common than many other nutrient deficiencies and is given its own section because it can significantly affect energy levels, exercise tolerance, hair health, and overall well-being.

During weight loss, especially with GLP-RA medications, iron intake may decrease because people eat less overall and/or avoid iron-rich foods. This can cause you to feel symptoms like fatigue or nausea. Iron deficiency can also worsen feelings of weakness or exhaustion, which may interfere with physical activity and long-term weight-loss success.

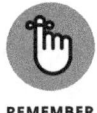

REMEMBER

The information in this section is meant to help you understand what iron deficiency anemia is and what your doctor may discuss with you if it is identified, not to replace personalized medical advice. Always review lab results and treatment options with your healthcare provider to determine what is appropriate for your individual health needs.

Iron deficiency anemia is commonly treated with over-the-counter oral iron supplements, such as ferrous sulfate or iron polysaccharide. Ferrous sulfate is inexpensive and widely used, but it can cause side effects like constipation, nausea, and stomach upset. Iron polysaccharide is gentler on the stomach and may be better tolerated, although it's often more expensive. Sometimes, your insurance may deny covering this iron formulation, but you can purchase it over the counter.

TECHNICAL STUFF

A key player in how your body absorbs iron is a hormone called **hepcidin** which is produced by the liver. Hepcidin controls iron levels by regulating how much iron can move from the food sources in your gut into your bloodstream. When hepcidin levels are high, iron becomes trapped inside cells of the gut. This significantly reduces how much iron enters the blood. When hepcidin levels are low, more dietary iron can be absorbed and released into the bloodstream for red blood cell production. Hepcidin levels rise in response to inflammation, infection, or high iron stores and fall when iron levels are low or the body needs to make more red blood cells. This regulation helps protect the body from iron overload, but in chronic inflammation or certain metabolic conditions, elevated hepcidin can unintentionally contribute to iron deficiency by limiting iron absorption.

Research has shown that taking oral iron once every 48 hours — not daily — may lead to better absorption and fewer side effects by allowing hepcidin levels to decrease between doses.

TIP

To improve iron absorption, take iron with a vitamin C–rich food such as orange juice, citrus fruits, kiwi, strawberries, tomatoes, or broccoli, and avoid coffee, tea, or calcium-rich foods at the same time, as they can interfere with absorption.

Maintaining Success: How to Keep the Weight Off

Losing weight is only half the battle. You may discover that the task of keeping the weight off is where the real work begins. Maintaining success means you must create habits, routines, and mindset shifts that make your healthier weight the new normal, not just a temporary milestone.

In the context of GLP-RA treatment, the maintenance phase means you have reached your goal total body weight loss while remaining on a stable, unchanging dose of medication. It also means your weight has remained steady without meaningful regain for at least six months, indicating that healthy habits and medication effects are working together to sustain your results.

Discontinuing your medication

Deciding when and how to discontinue a GLP-RA medication is an important step in the weight-loss journey and should always be done with medical guidance. Timing matters because these medications help regulate appetite, satiety, and eating behavior, and stopping them too early or abruptly can make it difficult to maintain weight loss. There is strong evidence showing that most people regain some or all of the weight once GLP-RA medications are stopped, especially if lifestyle habits are not firmly established. For this reason, stopping medication is generally not recommended unless there is a clear medical reason or a carefully planned transition strategy in place.

That said, the dietary, lifestyle, and habit changes you have built during treatment may strengthen your ability to maintain your goal weight. For some people, this creates an opportunity to reduce the medication dose rather than discontinue it entirely, while continuing to support appetite control and weight stability. Obesity is a chronic condition, and GLP-RA medications often function best as part of a long-term, individualized treatment plan.

If you and your doctor decide that stopping or reducing medication is appropriate, the process should be deliberate and personalized. The considerations below can help guide that discussion and reduce the risk of rapid weight regain.

Talk to your doctor about tapering your weight-loss meds when:

>> **You've maintained weight loss for six to twelve months.** In this context, maintenance means you have reached your target total body weight loss and your weight has remained stable, without meaningful regain, while on a steady dose of medication. Some clinicians may prefer that you are slightly below your goal weight before tapering, recognizing that a small amount of rebound can occur. This is one reason tapering is gradual and closely monitored rather than all at once.

>> **You've built sustainable habits.** This may include eating regular, balanced meals with adequate protein and fiber, engaging in consistent physical activity, managing stress, prioritizing sleep, and responding to hunger and fullness cues more reliably. These habits help support weight stability and reduce reliance on medication alone. Your doctor may look for evidence that these behaviors are consistent even during periods of stress or schedule disruption.

>> **You're no longer getting added benefit.** This can mean that appetite suppression has plateaued, weight has been stable for an extended period, or dose increases no longer produce additional weight loss or symptom improvement. It does not mean the medication has stopped working entirely, but rather that you may be at a point where a lower dose could provide the same benefit. Your doctor will help assess this based on weight trends, appetite signals, side effects, and overall quality of life.

REMEMBER

You will likely regain weight if you stop your GLP-RA medication too soon. Don't rush it. (See Chapter 2 for more information on the science of weight regain after stopping GLP-RAs.)

Preventing rebound weight gain

In clinical trials of GLP-1 receptor agonists like semaglutide, participants who stopped treatment regained about two-thirds of their prior weight loss over the following year. This rebound effect occurs because the medication's appetite-suppressing and metabolic benefits disappear. When appetite suppression is lost, your ability to maintain the same calorie deficit without substantial lifestyle changes can become nearly impossible. These findings highlight the importance of ongoing behavioral support, dietary adjustments, and regular physical activity when the medication is stopped to preserve long-term results.

TIP

When critical harmonizing body processes — appetite control, fullness signals, blood sugar, metabolism, muscle, sleep, stress, and daily movement — are breached, weight regain becomes very likely. Weight-loss medications support many of these systems, but your body may push back when medication is reduced or stopped. That is why habits matter so much during this stage. The goal is to keep these systems balanced. When they work together, maintaining weight is easier. When they do not, regain is more likely. The strategies below help keep these systems working together after medication. The goal is to support these systems together so they stay balanced. When they work in sync, your weight is easier to maintain. When one or more fall out of rhythm, regain becomes more likely. The strategies below are designed to help keep these processes working together after medication.

To avoid weight regain after you stop taking medication, follow some of these practical strategies:

>> **Ask ChatGPT.** AI tools can help you think through challenges as they come up. You can use them to plan meals, adjust routines, or problem solve when progress feels harder. They can also help you reflect on patterns and stay consistent when motivation dips. For more on using AI, check out the section earlier in this chapter, "Using AI prompts effectively."

>> **Weigh yourself weekly (not daily).** Weighing one time per week allows you to catch small increases early and adjust your habits before they snowball. Weighing daily, on the other hand, can be discouraging because weight normally changes from day to day due to fluids, digestion, and hormones. Weekly weighing supports awareness without obsession.

>> **Keep using apps — even if you're maintaining.** Keep using tracking tools, meal plans, or activity routines that helped you lose weight, even after you reach your goal because the apps help you notice small changes before they become bigger problems and keep healthy habits front of mind.

>> **Stay active with a routine you enjoy.** Enjoyable movement is easier to stick with long term. When you like what you are doing, you are more likely to keep showing up. Trying new activities can also keep things fresh and prevent boredom. Movement should fit your life and change as your interests and schedule change.

>> **Practice mindful eating.** Mindful eating means paying attention while you eat. You notice hunger, fullness, taste, and satisfaction. This helps you stop eating when you are comfortably full instead of eating out of habit or distraction. Over time, this supports better appetite control and prevents gradual overeating.

>> **Get plenty of sleep.** Sleep plays a major role in weight regulation. Too little sleep can increase hunger, cravings, and stress while lowering energy and motivation. Consistent, quality sleep helps balance hormones that control appetite and supports better decision-making during the day. The American Academy of Sleep Medicine recommends seven or more hours of sleep per night for adults.

>> **Catch weight creep of 2 to 3 pounds early.** A small gain is often the first sign that routines are slipping. This is a warning sign, not a failure. Early means noticing the change within a few weeks, not months or years. Making small adjustments at this stage is much easier than trying to reverse a larger regain later.

Establishing your maintenance mindset

Weight loss that lasts isn't only about what GLP-RA you take, which foods you eat, or how much you move. It's also about how you think and where you find comfort, reward, and fulfillment. Many people already begin to shift away from using food as their main source of stress relief or pleasure during weight loss, and this becomes even more important during maintenance. Mindfulness helps you stay aware of your choices and your body without judgment while also helping you notice fear and anxiety about regaining weight before those feelings take over. Learning to address those fears directly, rather than ignoring them or letting them drive your behavior, is a key part of staying on track long term.

Finding fulfillment outside of food

Finding fulfillment outside of food means training your brain to seek rewards beyond eating. This can feel insurmountable at first, but with time and dedication new passions can breed better habits for a fulfilling and healthy life. This pattern shift in finding fulfillment outside of food includes engaging your senses, connecting with others, pursuing passions, serving a purpose, and savoring simple, special moments. Activities like hiking, photography, learning a new skill, helping someone, or mindfully enjoying nature can create real joy and meaning. Over time, these experiences begin to replace food as the default source of comfort or celebration.

Fulfillment can come from creativity, connection, and caring for your mind and body. Hobbies like gardening, painting, writing, or music build skill and a sense of mastery, while relationships, community involvement, and helping others create a deeper, lasting satisfaction through connection. Mindful presence, such as savoring a cup of coffee or noticing the beauty around you, helps you feel more grounded to earth. Movement, rest, and small purposeful goals also support emotional wellbeing and reinforce that food is fuel, not the center of every reward.

Using mindfulness to stay on track

Mindfulness means staying attuned to your thoughts, feelings, and body without judgment. Mindfulness works by interrupting automatic eating patterns, lowering stress-driven food intake, and promoting healthier food choices. Mindfulness may be especially valuable to you during or after you have stopped using weight-loss drugs, because it helps you maintain behavior changes that prevent rebound weight gain.

You can practice mindfulness in simple, practical ways. Slow down while eating by putting your fork down between bites and checking in with your hunger and fullness. Eat without distractions when possible, such as turning off screens or stepping away from your phone. Pause before eating and ask yourself whether you are hungry, stressed, bored, or tired, and choose your response intentionally.

Mindfulness also extends beyond meals. Taking a few deep breaths during stressful moments can reduce the urge to eat reactively. Paying attention to how food makes you feel afterward helps guide future choices. Over time, these small practices become habits, like training in sports, and help you stay grounded and confident in maintenance.

TIP

Research suggests that mindfulness techniques can support weight loss and help sustain weight maintenance. These self-regulation techniques enhance your awareness of hunger, and fullness cues and can build coping mechanisms to avoid over and binge-eating. This scientific evidence shows that mindfulness-based approaches can lead to small but meaningful weight loss and fewer episodes of binge eating. Importantly, these benefits tend to last even after the program ends.

If this concept is new to you, and you have no idea where to begin or how to incorporate this practice into your routine, try:

>> Short, guided breathing exercises that last two to five minutes using the UCLA Mindful Awareness Research Center five-minute breathing meditation, Cleveland Clinic box breathing, or the three-minute breathing space

>> Basic mindfulness books or introductory articles focused on eating awareness including *Mindful Eating* (Shambhala 2017) by Jan Chozen Bays, *Eat What You Love, Love What You Eat* (Am I Hungry? Publishing 2020) by Michelle May, or introductory mindful eating articles from Harvard Health Publishing

>> Working with a counselor, coach, or dietitian who incorporates mindfulness into care, such as a registered dietitian trained in mindful eating, a behavioral health therapist using cognitive behavioral therapy with mindfulness, or a certified health coach focused on stress management (see Chapter 4 for more details on these types of teammates for your weight-loss journey)

If you need assistance with maintaining mindfulness, these online tools can teach you to pause before emotional eating, to reduce stress, and to stay grounded and connected to your goals:

>> **Mindfulness apps** like Headspace, Calm, and Eat Right Now

>> **Podcasts,** such as "The Mindful Minute" and "Mindful Muslim Podcast," for culturally tailored content

>> Guided meditation videos on YouTube

Addressing the fear and anxiety of rebounding

Fear of regaining weight is very common. Many people have seen weight come back after loss. Others may have experienced this themselves in the past. This fear can create constant worry and pressure.

Anxiety about rebound often leads to all-or-nothing thinking. A small change on the scale can feel like failure. This can lead to stress, restriction, or emotional eating. Stress makes maintenance harder, not easier.

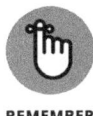

REMEMBER

The goal is not to eliminate fear. The goal is to respond to it in a healthier way. Structure and awareness help you feel more in control. Confidence builds when you see that small changes work.

Here are some tips to help control your fears:

>> Expect small weight changes and remind yourself this is normal.

>> Focus on habits you can control instead of the number on the scale.

>> Make a simple plan for early weight creep.

>> Use support tools when anxiety increases.

MINDFULNESS-BASED EATING AWARENESS TRAINING (MB-EAT)

Mindfulness-Based Eating Awareness Training (MB-EAT) is a structured, evidence-based program that helps individuals develop greater awareness of hunger, satiety, emotions, and environmental triggers that influence eating behaviors. It is typically delivered through guided group classes, workshops, or clinical programs led by trained facilitators, and can also be accessed through online courses or health system–based wellness programs. MB-EAT teaches practical skills such as mindful eating practices, slowing down during meals, and recognizing emotional versus physical hunger. By improving self-regulation and reducing mindless or stress-driven eating, MB-EAT can support sustainable weight loss and long-term weight management success.

3

Dealing with Unique Weight-Loss Situations

Learn how weight-loss medications are used across different ages, body types, and medical conditions.

See how clinicians approach treatment in women, men, older adults, and younger patients, and how chronic illnesses like diabetes, heart disease, or fatty liver can shape your plan.

Dive into the challenges that can appear at any stage such as your plateaus, insurance issues, shortages, side effects, or switching medications, and learn how to navigate each one of these obstacles confidently.

Discover what to do if medications fall short and how to use alternative strategies to keep your momentum.

Chapter **7**

Addressing Weight Loss for Various Populations

O besity-management looks different for every person, but certain populations require more individualized care. Factors, such as biology, life stage, social environment, and emotional health, all shape how your weight is gained, lost, and maintained. For example, women across their lifespan face unique hormonal and metabolic changes that influence their treatment needs, while children require family-centered strategies that focus on growth, development, and long-term health rather than rapid weight loss. Older adults need plans that protect muscle mass, preserve independence, and address common nutrient deficiencies, while people living with serious comorbid conditions require more careful personalized nutrition plans and specific medication adjustments to manage weight safely and effectively.

In this chapter, we address these unique populations. Not only do we highlight exactly what makes them unique, but we offer special guidance and support tailored specifically for each one.

Examining How GLP-RAs Impact Women's Health

Women often notice changes in their weight and metabolism at different stages of life, and it can feel confusing when the things that used to work stop working. During the childbearing years, factors like pregnancy, postpartum recovery, breastfeeding, and sleep disruption can all affect weight. Hormonal changes, stress, and less time for self-care can also play a role. During perimenopause and menopause, the body experiences natural shifts in estrogen and progesterone. These shifts can make weight loss feel harder than it used to be. Many women talk about gaining weight around the belly, feeling more tired, and noticing that their usual habits do not give the same results.

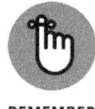

REMEMBER

This is not just in your head. Studies show that estrogen decline can lower metabolic rate, increase fat storage, and change how your body uses insulin. These changes can make weight-loss medications feel even more helpful because the medicines can support appetite control and metabolic regulation during a time when the body feels like it is working against you.

Understanding GLP-RAs in your childbearing years

The childbearing years come with unique challenges that affect weight and health. Pregnancy, postpartum recovery, breastfeeding, sleep loss, stress, and changing routines all affect appetite, metabolism, and energy. Hormones such as estrogen, progesterone, prolactin, cortisol, and insulin change during this time. These changes affect how the body stores fat, uses energy, and signals hunger. Sleep loss and stress can raise cortisol. Higher cortisol can increase appetite and promote weight gain. Many women gain weight with each pregnancy, and this weight can be hard to lose while caring for young children. These factors can make it feel like your body is working against you.

For women who are overweight or obese and want to become pregnant, GLP-RAs may be considered before conception, not during pregnancy. Obesity before pregnancy increases the risk of problems for both mother and baby, including gestational diabetes and blood sugar instability in the newborn. Babies born to mothers with obesity are more likely to have low blood sugars after delivery because of increases in their mother's insulin exposure to them during pregnancy. Losing weight before pregnancy can reduce these risks and support a healthier start for the baby.

GLP-RAs can be used as a tool to support weight loss before trying to conceive, alongside nutrition and lifestyle changes. Most women should give themselves enough time on medication to achieve meaningful and stable weight loss and to practice maintenance habits before pregnancy. This often means several months rather than weeks, followed by stopping the medication and allowing the body time to adjust before conception. GLP-RAs are not used during pregnancy, so planning ahead is important.

There is strong evidence that weight loss before pregnancy improves fertility and pregnancy outcomes. Weight loss can improve ovulation, hormone balance, and insulin sensitivity, making it easier to become pregnant. It also lowers the risk of gestational diabetes, high blood pressure, cesarean delivery, and complications for the baby. Preparing your body before pregnancy is one of the most powerful steps you can take to support a healthy pregnancy and birth.

REMEMBER

If you are taking a GLP-RA medication and are planning to become pregnant, you should stop taking the medication at least two months before attempting to conceive due to potential risks to the developing fetus. If you are thinking about becoming pregnant or are in a physically active relationship while on GLP-RAs, then you should consult with your doctor immediately. But don't worry: You have options. Contraceptive options, recommended by the American College of Obstetrics and Gynecology, can simultaneously help you plan and prevent pregnancy while optimizing your weight-loss journey while taking GLP-RAs. These options include long-acting reversible contraceptives (LARCs) like:

>> Hormonal intrauterine devices (IUD)s like Mirena and Kyleena

>> The copper IUD ParaGard

>> The arm implant, Nexplanon

WARNING

Weight-loss medications should not be used during pregnancy. If you are trying to conceive, you should talk with your doctor about stopping your medication before trying. GLP-RA medications have not been proven safe for a developing baby, and most guidelines recommend stopping these medicines at least two months before trying to get pregnant. There is evidence taken from animal studies which have shown potential negative effects on fetal development, including reduced fetal growth and birth defects when the fetus is exposed to GLP-RAs or other weight-loss medications in the womb.

REMEMBER

If you become pregnant while taking a GLP-1, you should notify your doctor right away. This is not a time to panic, but it is a time to stop the medication and switch focus toward healthy eating habits, prenatal vitamins, and safe prenatal care. After pregnancy, your doctor can help you decide when to restart medication if it is still part of your plan.

Using GLP-RAs during perimenopause and menopause

As estrogen levels drop, the risk for high blood pressure, high cholesterol, and type 2 diabetes goes up. This is why so many women feel like weight is no longer a cosmetic issue but a bonafide health issue. Research shows that visceral fat often increases during menopause, and this type of fat raises the risk for heart disease. Even women who keep their weight steady can notice changes in where fat settles. This fat tends to accumulate around the abdomen which is specifically linked to higher metabolic risk. These changes explain why even small amounts of weight loss during menopause can make a big difference in your future heart and metabolic health.

GLP-RAs work well for women during perimenopause and menopause because they directly help the systems that menopause can disrupt. These medicines support blood sugar balance, lower appetite, and help reduce fat around the abdomen. In fact, women in perimenopause and menopause lose weight on GLP-RA medications at similar rates to younger adults.

In large trials, GLP-RA medicines like semaglutide and tirzepatide produced meaningful weight loss in women older than over 45 years. The typical weight loss in these studies ranged from 12 percent to more than 20 percent TBWL depending on the medication and the dose. Women also showed improvements in blood pressure, blood sugar, and cholesterol. These results matter because this stage of life is a time when cardiometabolic risk starts rising, and even modest weight loss can reduce your long-term complications.

In some studies, insulin sensitivity in postmenopausal women is even improved. Many women report that GLP-RAs give them back a sense of control over hunger and cravings when their hormones feel unpredictable. These medications do not replace hormones, but they often work well and safely alongside hormone therapy when your doctor thinks both are appropriate.

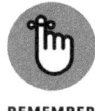

REMEMBER

GLP-RA medications do not increase estrogen or progesterone. They do not behave like hormone therapy, and they do not fix low hormone levels. What they do is help smooth out the metabolic impact that falling hormones create. Research shows that GLP-1 medications can lower inflammation markers and improve insulin sensitivity, which are two things that often worsen as estrogen declines. Some small studies suggest GLP-1s may help with hot flashes because they influence blood vessel tone, but this is still early research. The main point is that GLP-RAs can support weight and metabolic health during menopause without affecting reproductive hormones.

Checking Out Children's Weight Loss

Parents often want to help their kids develop healthy habits, but weight loss in children must be handled carefully. A parent may talk with a child's doctor if growth patterns change or if weight seems high for age and height. Concerns may also come up if a child shows health issues linked to weight, such as high blood pressure, high blood sugar, or sleep problems. Doctors routinely track height, weight, and BMI over time to look for concerning trends.

In most cases, the first step is not weight loss but supporting healthy behaviors for the whole family. This includes nutrition, movement, sleep, and emotional well-being. Some children may need more support if weight-related health risks are present and habits alone are not enough. Older children and teens with ongoing obesity may be evaluated for additional options under medical guidance. The goal is always to protect health and development, not to focus on a number on the scale. This section helps parents understand when and how to start these conversations safely with their child's doctor.

WARNING

Children are still growing, so your goal to assist your child should be better health and gentler weight change rather than strict weight loss. Doctors focus on growth charts and look at patterns over time (averaged as grams per day) rather than isolated numbers.

Exploring key guidelines for children's weight loss

The 2023 American Academy of Pediatrics Clinical Practice Guideline emphasizes that childhood obesity is a complex, systemic disease influenced by environmental, social, and genetic factors. Understanding that obesity in children is very different from adults is important because children are still growing physically and developmentally. Their bodies need adequate nutrition to support brain development, bone growth, and puberty, which means weight loss must be approached carefully. Children also have different hormone patterns and metabolic needs that change with age. In addition, eating behaviors, activity levels, and health habits in children are strongly shaped by family, school, and environment rather than individual choice alone. For these reasons, treatment in children focuses on healthy growth and long-term health, not rapid or restrictive weight loss. The approach to alter the trajectory of abnormal growth in pediatric obesity requires a comprehensive, family-centered treatment approach. For more discussion on this guideline, see Chapter 12.

Because children are still growing, the goal is not rapid weight loss or strict diet-ing. Instead, care focuses on supporting healthy growth while reducing future health risks. This is why the American Academy of Pediatrics emphasizes early screening, family involvement, and medical guidance rather than waiting until problems become severe. The approach is gradual, structured, and matched to a child's age, development, and health needs. The guidelines below reflect this framework and show how treatment becomes more intensive only when simpler, supportive steps are not enough.

These recommendations outline when lifestyle-based care is appropriate and when additional medical tools may be considered. They also explain why deci-sions are guided by age, growth patterns, and health risks rather than weight alone. Understanding this framework helps parents see how each option fits into a stepwise plan. (See the later section, "Figuring out if your child is a candidate for GLP-RAs," to see whether your child may be a candidate for any of these approaches.)

Overall, the guideline underscores the need for proactive screening, early intervention, and coordinated care led by pediatricians and primary health care providers to prevent long-term complications. Some of the key points of this guideline include:

» Children ages 6 and older should be referred to intensive, family-based behavioral treatment programs, with the strongest evidence for programs providing at least 26 hours of contact over 3 to 12 months.

» Weight-loss medicines may be considered beginning at age 12 for those with BMI at or above the 95th percentile.

» Bariatric surgery may be appropriate for those age 13 and older with extreme obesity.

The guideline recommends early evaluation for related conditions using labs such as fasting glucose, HbA1c, liver function tests, lipid panels, and blood pressure monitoring. Polysomnography (sleep study) should be considered if your child snores or if sleep apnea is suspected.

Figuring out if your child is a candidate for GLP-RAs

Parents often start this conversation when they notice that healthy habits alone are not improving their child's weight or health. This may include continued weight gain, rising BMI over time, or the development of health concerns such as high blood sugar, high blood pressure, fatty liver disease, or sleep apnea. A doctor will review your child's growth history, age, BMI percentile, and overall health, not just the number on the scale. They will also ask about daily habits, family routines, mental health, and how previous lifestyle-based treatments have worked.

TIP

GLP-RAs are generally considered for adolescents who meet age and BMI criteria and who have obesity-related health risks. They are not usually used for children who are still responding well to lifestyle changes alone. If a child is just under the cutoff, the focus often remains on intensive family-based programs and close follow up. Readiness to take medication, ability to follow the treatment plan, and family support also matter. If medication is not appropriate, the doctor will help guide other safe and effective options to support your child's health.

Getting to know child-friendly weight-loss treatments

Treating obesity early is the most effective way to prevent the lifelong burden of severe metabolic disease in children. Like adults, children can benefit from a lot of the same interventions. Some children benefit from structured nutrition support, family-based activity changes, and behavioral therapy. But others might require weight-loss medication.

TIP

Five weight-loss medications are approved for adolescents: orlistat, Qsymia, Wegovy, Mounjaro, and Saxenda. GLP-RA medications, like Wegovy and Saxenda, are approved for children age 12 and older with obesity, but medication use in younger patients such as these requires close supervision because their bodies are still developing.

There are certainly instances during which other medications, like metformin, are used to treat obesity in children. Metform is a drug which serves as a sensitizer of your body's cells to insulin. Its main action is to reduce glucose production in the liver, which lowers fasting blood sugar. Metformin also improves insulin sensitivity, helping muscles and other tissues use glucose more effectively. In research trials, metformin has been shown to decrease BMI significantly more in children than either placebo or lifestyle management. When this drug is used in obesity, even in the absence of a diagnosis of diabetes for your child, it is being applied "off label."

GETTING THE FACTS ON OFF-LABEL USE

Off-label does not equate to experimental. The Federal Food, Drug, and Cosmetic Act, originally passed in 1938, does not, however, limit the way a physician may use an approved drug. Once a product has been approved for marketing, a physician may prescribe it for uses or in treatment regimens or patient populations that are not included in approved labeling, such as children. Such unapproved or, more precisely, *unlabeled* uses may be appropriate and rational in certain circumstances.

In fact, these prescribing practices may reflect approaches to drug therapy that have been extensively reported in medical literature. In much the same way, other GLP-RA drugs such as tirzepatide may be prescribed in children, but when this occurs, it's being conducted in an off label-fashion because tirzepatide is not FDA-approved for patients under age 18 years. When this occurs, ensure that your child is managed by a skilled pediatric obesity medicine specialist. The most important step is to involve a pediatrician who understands obesity medicine and can guide the family toward safe and realistic goals. Preferably this pediatrician is board-certified in obesity medicine. See Chapter 4 for more information on building a healthcare team around your child.

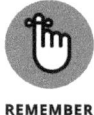

REMEMBER

The diagnosis of severe pediatric obesity is rising quickly, and its health consequences are profound. Children with obesity experience early onset of insulin resistance, metabolic syndrome, metabolic dysfunction–associated steatotic liver disease (MASLD), and diabetes at higher rates than adults with the same BMI. Diet changes and food policy alone cannot reverse extreme obesity once it is established. The data show that the longer obesity persists in childhood, the harder it becomes to treat. When this occurs, it is more likely for your child to suffer major, preventable complications during their lifetime. This makes early intervention critical.

THE NEED FOR BETTER-SUPPORTED OBESITY CARE IN CHILDREN

Children with obesity deserve care that is accessible, affordable, and guided by medical experts. Obesity is a chronic disease, not a failure of effort or parenting. Many families struggle to find care that goes beyond basic advice and provides real support. When treatment is delayed, health risks such as diabetes, high blood pressure, and liver disease become more likely. Early treatment helps protect a child's physical health and emotional well-being. The bottom line is that treating obesity early is the most effective way to prevent lifelong metabolic disease.

Here are some reasonable steps parents can take

- Ask your child's pediatrician for referral to a comprehensive pediatric weight management or obesity clinic

- Discuss whether medication options, including GLP-RAs, may be appropriate now or in the future

- Advocate for insurance coverage of family-based programs, nutrition counseling, and obesity medications

Rare, genetic forms

Children can suffer from some rare, genetic forms of obesity. These include: Prader–Willi syndrome, proopiomelanocortin (POMC) deficiency, proprotein convertase subtilisin/kexin type 1 (PCSK1) deficiency, leptin receptor (LEPR) deficiency, and Bardet–Biedl syndrome. This section details more information on these rare conditions and medications that may help.

TIP

If you are concerned that your child has one of these conditions, you should seek the care of a general pediatrician for a possible referral to a genetics, pediatric endocrinology, or pediatric obesity medicine specialist.

Medication to treat Prader–Willi syndrome (PWS)

Prader-Willi syndrome is a rare genetic disorder characterized by poor muscle tone, insatiable appetite leading to obesity, intellectual disability, and hormonal deficiencies due to hypothalamic dysfunction. PWS is caused by the loss of function of paternally inherited genes on chromosome 15q11-q13. The hormonal dysfunction resulting from PWS tends to cause hyperphagia, the symptom of always eating, always feeling hungry, and never being satiated by food.

ARD-101 is a novel, oral small-molecule drug developed by Aardvark Therapeutics to treat hyperphagia. The drug works by activating multiple bitter taste receptors (TAS2R) in the gut, which then stimulate the release of key hormones such as cholecystokinin (CCK) and GLP-1/GLP-2 which should make the patient feel satiated.

A Phase 2 study completed in September 2024 (NCT05153434) enrolled adults with PWS. It met its research study goals, with 11 of 12 participants showing reduced hyperphagia scores after 28 days with far fewer side effects reported than other GLP-RAs with active FDA approval.

The ongoing Phase 3 HERO Trial (NCT06828861), which started December 2024 and is expected to complete in April 2026, tests ARD-101 against placebo in individuals aged 13 and older. The early study results have shown that so far, ARD-101 appears "well tolerated" and may significantly reduce intense hunger in PWS.

Inherited and genetic forms of obesity

In very rare cases, obesity can be due to inherited reasons or other genetic mutations where your body may not produce the receptor to signal fullness after a meal, including

» POMC deficiency (affecting approximately 1 in 1 to 5 million people): POMC deficiency can present as obesity in the first year of life accompanied by pale complexion, fatigue, and lack of response to mealtimes with near constant hunger (hyperphagia).

» PCSK1 deficiency (affecting approximately 1 in 250,000 to 1 million): PCSK1 Deficiency is characterized by early-onset obesity, frequent diarrhea or malabsorption, and episodes of low blood sugar (hypoglycemia), particularly in infancy. These children may also have hormone deficiencies affecting growth and development. Families should seek care if a child is gaining weight rapidly and experiencing digestive issues or signs of hormonal imbalance.

» LEPR deficiency (affecting approximately 1 in 1 to 3 million): LEPR deficiency leads to severe obesity early in life due to intense, unrelenting hunger. Children may never feel full and show delayed or absent puberty (hypogonadism). Some may also have a weakened immune system. Parents should be concerned if their child becomes very overweight early on and seems constantly hungry, especially if puberty is delayed or absent.

» Bardet–Biedl syndrome (affecting approximately 1 in 100,000 to 160,000 in the general population; incidence can be higher in certain isolated or consanguineous populations [e.g., Middle Eastern, Amish], where it may reach 1 in 13,000): Bardet-Biedl Syndrome (BBS) involves a broader range of symptoms including childhood obesity, extra fingers or toes (polydactyly), progressive vision loss (starting with night blindness), kidney problems, and developmental delays. Hormonal or genital anomalies are also common. If a child is obese and also has visual, cognitive, or physical abnormalities, evaluation for BBS should be considered.

For those patients with one of these rare conditions, there is hope on the weight-loss journey! Setmelanotide is a melanocortin-4 receptor (MC4R) agonist. The MC4R pathway plays a critical role in regulating appetite and body weight. In people with genetic conditions like POMC, LEPR, or PCSK1 deficiency, this pathway is disrupted, leading to uncontrolled hunger (hyperphagia) and severe obesity from a young age.

Setmelanotide is FDA-approved for chronic weight management in patients with POMC, PCSK1, LEPR deficiency, and Bardet-Biedl syndrome (BBS). Setmelanotide is a once-daily subcutaneous injection. This medication will not be helpful in patients without one of these specific genetic conditions or for your general weight-loss journey. Setmelanotide should only be selected in close consultation with a physician skilled in the management of these rare conditions such as a pediatric obesity medicine specialist or geneticist.

Focusing on Geriatric Weight Loss

Successful weight loss in older adults depends on preserving muscle mass through resistance training, ensuring adequate protein and nutrient intake, and using safe, gradual lifestyle changes. Oftentimes, negative lifelong habits are difficult to overcome, and medication management or bariatric surgical intervention may be indicated to help you achieve your goals. Consult your obesity medicine specialist to help determine which would be the best option for you. Thankfully, GLP-RAs appear safe in geriatric patients, with little to no drug-to-drug interactions that might cause toxicity with your other medications. When these fundamentals are in place, obese geriatric patients can improve mobility, maintain independence, and experience meaningful gains in quality of life.

Research shows that GLP-RA medicines can improve diabetes control and heart health in older adults. You can read Chapter 12 to see that multiple scientific groups focused on obesity care recommend the use of weight-loss medication and/or bariatric surgery with no upper age limit or cut off.

Grasping your unique needs as an older adult

Older adults have unique macro- and micronutrient needs, and two major markers of malnutrition in this population include:

>> **Sarcopenia:** A condition marked by a progressive loss of skeletal muscle mass and strength.

>> **Cachexia:** A condition that involves more complex metabolic changes caused by underlying illnesses such as cancer, end-stage renal disease, or congestive heart failure. Cachexia results in muscle loss with or without fat loss.

The goal for an older adult is to preserve normal nutrition and avoid these complicated states if using GLP-RAs. Because these conditions can develop subtly and worsen health outcomes, early identification is essential. Several screening tools exist to help detect risk, and the Mini Nutritional Assessment (MNA) is one of the most widely used for assessing malnutrition and undernutrition in older adults.

Key to management of obesity in geriatric patients is the fundamental understanding that your nutritional requirements shift as you age because most become somewhat *hypometabolic*, which means you may require less energy or calories each day to sustain health.

The greatest concern is that if older patients who are obese start on the heavy end of the weight spectrum and then they initiate GLP-RAs and rapidly uptitrate, it may swing the pendulum to the other side and miss the mark entirely! This could cause preventable complications of sarcopenia and cachexia and negatively affect your health.

Fitting in the physical side of weight loss

Weight-loss goals in older adults should prioritize strength, safety, and overall health rather than rapid changes on the scale because as you age, you lose muscle more easily. So unplanned weight loss can cause your body to be frail. So your plan should always include not only intentional nutrition but also resistance strength exercises to maintain independence and mobility. Resistance training for geriatric patients can start with these simple exercises:

>> Chair-assisted squats, which help build leg strength and improve balance.

>> Light dumbbells or resistance bands can be used for bicep curls and overhead presses to maintain upper-body muscle mass.

>> Seated rows with a resistance band strengthens the back and supports good posture, which often declines with age.

>> Wall push-ups are another safe option that build chest and arm strength without placing heavy strain on the joints.

Losing Weight When You Have Comorbidities

Your body is a complex interplay between multiple systems, and comorbid conditions can negatively impact other facets of your overall health. Comorbidities are medical conditions that occur at the same time as another condition, such as obesity. When you have one or more comorbidities, your body systems affect each other in complex ways. A condition like diabetes, sleep apnea, arthritis, or liver disease can make weight loss harder by changing hormones, energy use, appetite, or physical ability. The impact on weight loss depends on the specific comorbidity and how severe it is. The flip side is also true: Improvement in one condition can oftentimes help another. That is why weight loss for obesity causes a positive domino effect on many conditions leading to global life improvements.

Obesity is closely linked to many chronic diseases because excess fat drives inflammation, insulin resistance, and places immense strain on multiple organs. These changes can create a metabolic environment that resists weight loss. For example, obesity increases the risk of type 2 diabetes by making it harder for the body to use insulin, and severe insulin resistance can further slow weight loss. Weight loss can help reverse many of these changes. Losing weight improves how the body responds to insulin and helps lower blood sugar levels. As insulin sensitivity improves, the body is better able to use energy instead of storing it as fat. These improvements can also reduce inflammation and ease strain on organs, which can lead to better control of conditions like high blood pressure, fatty liver disease, and abnormal cholesterol. This is why weight loss for obesity can be a powerful, universal game changer for your overall health.

Detailing the consequences of comorbidities

Comorbid conditions may complicate your health. The encouraging news is that even modest, sustained weight loss can lead to meaningful improvements across many body systems. Lower weight can improve blood sugar, blood pressure, cholesterol, heart strain, and liver fat, which together support better long-term health and quality of life. Ultimately this can improve your long-term health and quality of life. In fact, in a recent, real-world study of more than 280,000 adults with obesity, GLP-1 medications were associated with 24 percent lower cardiovascular events, 36 percent lower kidney events, and 51 percent lower all-cause mortality compared with other obesity non-GLP-RA drugs. Mental-health outcomes also improved significantly, including lower depression, suicidal ideation, and substance-use disorders. Studies did not show a higher risk of pancreatitis or low blood sugar. Weight-loss medications appear to globally enhance health for patients with obesity.

These conditions can make your health more complicated and can make weight loss harder. They affect how your body controls hunger, energy use, and metabolism. They can also limit how active you feel or increase fatigue and stress. Together, these factors make losing weight more challenging than it would be otherwise. The breakdown below will help you better understand the impact of these other conditions on your weight and your overall health, and you will also see how GLP–RAs can serve as the key to correct some of these problems.

>> **Diabetes:** Obesity will increase your risk of developing type 2 diabetes by making it harder for the body to use insulin effectively, and severe insulin signaling impairment creates a metabolic state that makes weight loss more difficult. When this happens, excess calories are stored as fat, which means that the weight you gain will be harder to lose. Studies show that GLP-1 medications improve insulin sensitivity, lower blood sugar, and reduce the need for other diabetes medications.

>> **Congestive heart failure:** When you carry extra weight, this potentially worsens congestive heart failure by increasing cardiac workload and fluid retention. This can lead to shortness of breath, fatigue, and reduced ability to exercise, which limits calorie burn and makes weight loss harder. Heart failure also raises the risk of hospitalizations and early death. Research shows that GLP-1 medications reduce body weight and improve cardiovascular outcomes, leading to fewer heart-related events.

>> **Hypertension:** You may experience hypertension (high blood pressure) with obesity because excess adipose tissue raises resistance in your blood. High blood pressure strains the heart, kidneys, and brain and increases the risk of stroke and heart attack. It can also limit exercise tolerance and worsen fatigue, which interferes with weight-loss efforts. Studies show that GLP-1 medications lower blood pressure and reduce overall cardiovascular risk through weight loss and improved vascular health.

>> **Hyperlipidemia:** High cholesterol and triglycerides often accompany obesity, contributing to hyperlipidemia and plaque buildup in your arteries. This increases the risk of heart disease and stroke. Abnormal lipid levels also reflect underlying metabolic dysfunction, which makes weight loss more resistant. Research shows that GLP-1 medications improve lipid profiles, especially triglycerides, by improving insulin sensitivity and reducing fat mass.

>> **Metabolic dysfunction–associated steatotic liver disease (MASLD):** Fat accumulation in the liver can lead to MASLD (previously NAFLD), which may progress to fibrosis or cirrhosis, the condition in which the liver stops functioning properly. This creates a cycle that promotes further weight gain and metabolic disease. Over time, MASLD can progress to liver inflammation, scarring, or cirrhosis. Studies show that GLP-1 medications reduce liver fat and improve liver inflammation through sustained weight loss and better metabolic control.

>> **Renal disease:** Obesity also raises the risk of end-stage renal disease by damaging blood vessels and accelerating diabetic kidney injury due to excessive, chronically high blood pressures. Declining kidney function can cause fatigue, fluid retention, and medication limitations that complicate

weight loss. Kidney disease also increases the risk of heart disease and early mortality. Research shows that GLP-1 medications slow the progression of kidney disease and reduce kidney-related complications in people with obesity.

TECHNICAL
STUFF

People with diabetes and obesity tend to lose about half as much weight on GLP-1 therapy as those who are obese without diabetes. A new study showed that early, aggressive weight-loss treatment can lead to remission of type 2 diabetes. Patients who received weight-loss medication plus a high-protein diet and structured exercise had dramatically better outcomes than those on standard therapy. More than 86 percent of people with type 2 diabetes achieved remission, and over 73 percent of people with prediabetes returned to normal glucose.

Nailing the nutritional points

When you are taking weight-loss medications, nutrition plays an important role in how well they work. Choosing foods that support your specific health conditions can improve weight loss and reduce complications.

TIP

Specific nutrition choices for certain comorbid conditions can help control blood sugar, blood pressure, and inflammation while on GLP-RAs. This support helps your body respond better to medication and makes weight loss more effective and sustainable.

There are some key nutritional points worth your consideration which are disease specific:

>> **Diabetes:** Healthy eating for type 2 diabetes starts with reducing daily calories, choosing balanced meals, and aiming for gradual weight loss of about 5 to 10 percent. This can significantly improve your blood sugar and sometimes even lead to your diabetes remission. Most people benefit from choosing a macronutrient pattern with 45 to 60 percent carbohydrate, 10 to 20 percent protein, and less than 35 percent fat. You should try and limit your saturated fat intake to under 10 percent of your total calories and keep sodium below 6 grams of salt per day.

>> **Congestive heart failure (CHF):** This becomes mostly about monitoring your salt and fluid intake. Heart failure guidelines recommend keeping sodium intake below 6 grams of salt per day, and fluid restriction is often necessary, limited to about 1.5 to 2 liters (up to 2 quarts) per day depending on your symptoms and volume status. Research shows that following the DASH diet along with reducing salt intake can lower heart disease markers by 20 to 23 percent. Overall, the strongest evidence supports the DASH diet, with

both DASH and Mediterranean patterns offering meaningful cardiovascular benefits for patients with heart failure.

» **Hypertension:** The DASH diet has been shown to lower blood pressure in people without diabetes and in those with well-controlled diabetes. Be aware, the DASH diet improves blood pressure, but it does not typically lead to significant weight loss.

» **Hyperlipidemia:** Decreasing hyperlipidemia starts with adjusting the types and amounts of fats in your diet. Most guidelines recommend limiting saturated fat to less than 10 percent of total daily calories if you are obese. If you have hyperlipidemia and obesity, the goal may need to be for you to limit saturated fats to less than 5 to 6 percent of total calories. This usually means reducing culprit foods in your diet like fatty meats, full-fat dairy, butter, tropical oils, and ultra-processed foods. At the same time, increasing your intake of unsaturated fats, especially monounsaturated and omega-3–rich options such as olive oil, nuts, seeds, avocados, and fatty fish, can help lower LDL and triglycerides while supporting higher HDL levels. Cutting back on both refined carbohydrates and added sugars also improves triglycerides. Among dietary patterns, the Mediterranean diet consistently shows the strongest evidence for improving blood pressure, reducing triglycerides, raising HDL, and lowering cardiovascular risk.

» **MASLD/NAFLD:** Managing MASLD/NAFLD begins with understanding that this condition is driven by metabolic dysfunction, insulin resistance, and excess liver fat. Weight loss remains the most effective intervention recommended by current society guidelines. If you were to lose as little as 5 to 10 percent in body weight, you can significantly decrease liver fat, improve inflammation, and slow or reverse early fibrosis/scarring. New MASLD terminology emphasizes its metabolic roots, highlighting the need for lifestyle strategies that improve cardiometabolic health. Evidence also supports using Mediterranean-style eating patterns, which improve liver enzymes, reduce steatosis, and lower cardiovascular risk which is the leading cause of death in MASLD.

» **End-stage renal disease (ESRD):** A stage-4 chronic kidney disease diet focuses on lowering protein, phosphorus, potassium, and sodium to reduce kidney workload. These strategies aim to preserve your remaining kidney function. Patients are encouraged to choose low-potassium fruits and vegetables, limit high-phosphorus foods, and include high-quality protein sources in small amounts.

Chapter **8**

Navigating Medication Challenges

You may be one of the many people who struggle with obesity and encounter obstacles along their weight-loss journey. After trying diets, exercise routines, lifestyle changes, and possibly even therapy, medication options may feel like the final hope. So you don't make the decision to seek medical assistance in the form of weight-loss medication lightly. These medicines represent the key that might finally unlock lasting weight loss, but when the medications don't work, stop working, or cause side effects too severe to continue their use — a unique kind of frustration and uncertainty can follow.

Obesity is a complex, chronic condition influenced by biology, environment, psychology, and social factors. It's not simply the result of poor eating choices. Unfortunately, those struggling with obesity or the inability to lose weight often suffer from an unfair social stigma.

REMEMBER

When medications fail or cause side effects, the failure can compound the feeling of being stigmatized and cause an even more painful experience. It's not just a treatment that didn't work — it feels like yet another personal failure, even though it absolutely isn't.

But what comes next matters most. When medications don't work and you feel lost on your journey, you have options! Your weight-loss journey is far from hopeless. You have ways to navigate the road ahead that respect your experience, maintain your well-being, and offer real opportunities for healing and achievement of weight loss.

In this chapter, you discover some common reasons why weight-loss medications don't work for everyone, including genetic, metabolic, and lifestyle conditions that affect how the medications interact with your body. You can also take a look at adverse reactions and unpleasant side effects that can make taking a weight-loss medication not be the optimal choice for you.

Understanding Why Weight-Loss Medications May Fail

Before you dive into alternative approaches, you should understand why weight-loss medications might not work. These medications are promising and effective for some people, but they aren't miracle cures. We have to keep in mind, these drugs are designed to aid weight loss, hand-in-hand with diet and lifestyle changes. Even under ideal conditions, the average weight loss tends to be modest — typically 5 to 15 percent of your total body weight.

Common reasons for medication ineffectiveness

You can find several reasons that explain why the medication prescribed for you might not be effective:

>> **Genetics and metabolism:** Some bodies are simply more resistant to weight loss due to how they metabolize food, store fat, or regulate hormones like insulin and leptin.

>> **Underlying conditions:** Polycystic ovarian syndrome (PCOS), hypothyroidism, insulin resistance, and mental health issues, such as depression or binge eating disorder, can all undermine the effects of weight-loss drugs.

>> **Medication mismatch:** Not all weight-loss drugs work for everyone. What's effective for one person may do little for another. It is important for you to have a conversation with your doctor which designs a personalized weight-loss plan to your needs. (See Chapter 4 for more on choosing your healthcare team.)

>> **Medication counter-activity:** Some prescription medications can *counteract* (reduce effectiveness) of or increase your *body's metabolism* (speed up rate at which your body burns through) weight-loss drugs. (You can review Chapter 2 for a more in-depth discussion on mechanism of drug action.) Specifically, those medications include:

- *Opioids* — such as morphine, codeine, oxycodone, hydrocodone — can slow gastric emptying, potentially reducing the effectiveness of GLP-RAs.

- *Glucocorticoids/systemic steroids* such as Prednisone may increase blood glucose levels, counteracting the glucose-lowering effects of GLP-RAs that help you lose weight.

- *Diuretics* — such as chlorothiazide, furosemide, and spironolactone — can lead to dehydration and electrolyte imbalances, which may affect overall metabolic processes which must function optimally for weight loss.

- Certain *antiepileptic drugs* such as phenytoin and carbamazepine may induce liver enzymes, potentially increasing the metabolism of GLP-RAs.

- *Rifampin* is an antibiotic known to induce cytochrome P450 enzymes, which could lead to increased clearance of GLP-RAs.

>> **Tolerance or plateau:** Some people experience an initial, early drop in weight, only to plateau as the body adjusts to the medication. When this occurs, the medication is usually still working if you feel satisfied after meals and your cravings are under control. This early plateau phenomenon is manageable and very different from tolerance, which tends to present itself after sustained, long-term medication exposure. When this **plateau** occurs, dose escalation following the official drug titration schedule usually does the trick.

Signs and symptoms of **tolerance** may include increased hunger, feeling less full after regular meals, and slower weight loss despite the same drug dose. When tolerance is suspected, oftentimes you need to consider switching drug classes, for example, changing from semaglutide to tirzepatide (see Chapter 2 for a look at the various weight-loss drug classes).

>> **Side effects:** Nausea, fatigue, mood changes, and other side effects can make it impossible to continue treatment with a specific medication. In this case, you might consider altering your diet. Foods that are "mashable" with a fork and liquids may be easier for your stomach to digest and cause less nausea. In other instances, you may seek help from the anti-nausea medication, Ondansetron, also known as Zofran. You can typically make these small changes to your weight-loss journey regimen to great success. Rarely, you will find that the side effects of a medication are too great, making it feel impossible to continue your weight-loss drug. In those instances, you should follow our "Handling Adverse Reactions and Side Effects" section later in this chapter.

Focusing on the role of genetics and metabolism in weight loss

Recent, high-quality genetic research demonstrates that individual susceptibility to weight gain and metabolic efficiency is deeply rooted in your genetic makeup. These genetic factors control how the body processes energy, stores fat, regulates appetite, and responds to environmental cues such as physical activity.

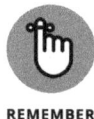

A genetic predisposition to obesity can make weight management more challenging, but it does not eliminate the effectiveness of lifestyle interventions. Understanding these genetic influences can lead to more personalized approaches to obesity prevention and treatment, ultimately improving health outcomes across populations.

Some of the most important genetic markers related to obesity include:

>> **FTO (fat mass and obesity-associated) gene:** FTO changes have been linked to increased appetite, higher caloric intake, and reduced satiety. Individuals with FTO types may be more prone to overeating and gaining weight.

>> **MC4R (melanocortin 4 receptor) gene:** The MC4R receptor is part of the melanocortin system, which influences feeding behavior and energy expenditure. It is primarily expressed in the brain, particularly in the hypothalamus, where it helps control hunger and satiety signals. Mutations can lead to a loss of function, resulting in increased appetite and reduced energy expenditure.

Other more global factors can affect your ability to lose weight. Two factors which may have a significant effect on this ability include:

>> *Polygenetics: The idea that a group of genes that interact additively to influence a phenotypic trait, such as slow metabolism, highly efficient energy storage, conversion of calories to fat*

Some people naturally have a slower metabolism due to inherited traits, making it more difficult for them to maintain or lose weight. Additionally, genes involved in fat oxidation, insulin sensitivity, and muscle composition can significantly impact how efficiently the body uses energy.

>> *Epigenetics: The study of how environmental factors influence gene expression*

Researchers have directly linked epigenetics to difficulty in achieving weight loss. For example, they've linked early life nutrition — such as for pre-term infants who are low birth weight or children who develop obesity early in life — to development of obesity in adulthood. Additional factors, such as stress and even sleep patterns, can alter how genes related to metabolism function throughout life.

TIP

Possessing genetic predisposition to obesity does not make weight loss impossible. But you may have to work harder to lose weight compared to others' efforts. Importantly, gene–environment interactions play a key role. Discuss these genetics-related concerns with your doctor.

Except in rare instances, such as children who have obesity, genetic screening is not indicated prior to starting weight-loss medications.

Lifestyle Factors and Medication Efficacy

GLP-RAs provide a valuable pharmacological tool for weight loss, but you must pair the medication with sustainable lifestyle habits like mindful eating, nutritious food choices, physical activity, proper hydration, sufficient sleep, and stress management. This will maximize its effects. These changes not only help achieve weight-loss goals more efficiently but also lay the foundation for long-term weight maintenance and improved overall health.

While GLP-RAs can be highly effective, the success of your weight loss is greatly enhanced when combined with the practical lifestyle changes mentioned. In this section, you find several evidence-based lifestyle factors that can support and accelerate weight loss while you also use GLP-RAs.

Mindful eating habits

GLP-RAs reduce appetite and slows gastric emptying, which naturally helps users feel full with less food. This effect can be optimized by practicing mindful eating. You should learn to listen to hunger cues, eat slowly, and avoid distractions like phones or television during meals. Eating more slowly gives GLP-RAs more time to work and helps prevent overeating. Portion control is also important, even if you're feeling less hungry. (See Chapter 5 for more tips on integrating these lifestyle choices and habit changes with your GLP-RA medicine.)

Balanced, nutrient-dense diet

Although GLP-RAs seek to decrease appetite, the quality of nutrients in your food still matters. Malnutrition is an underestimated complication of GLP-1 medications, especially as these drugs are prescribed more widely. Your reduced appetite and rapid weight loss can lead to unintended protein and micronutrient deficiencies, particularly in older adults and those already at nutritional risk. Your safest dietary choices emphasize whole, nutrient-dense foods such as lean proteins (chicken, tofu, fish), fiber-rich vegetables, whole grains, and healthy fats (avocados, olive oil, nuts). Protein helps preserve lean muscle mass during weight loss and enhances satiety. Fiber slows digestion, further supporting feelings of fullness.

You should minimize eating highly processed foods, sugary snacks, and refined carbohydrates because they can spike blood sugar and reduce the benefits of GLP-RAs. (See Chapter 5 for more information about reworking your diet.) Part of your vigilance is to spot and avoid ultra-processed foods. These foods have been clearly linked to the development of obesity, type 2 diabetes, and high blood pressure.

TIP

Here's how to spot those ultra-processed foods that you want to avoid:

>> **Inspect the nutrition label of the bag or a box that contains the food.** Granted, some healthy foods — such as frozen fruit — come in a bag but are not ultra-processed. But to make sure, turn over the bag or box and read the ingredients and nutrition label. Even safe, whole foods may have a short ingredient list, but if the list includes several chemical names that you do not know, this is a red flag.

>> **Look for tell-tale wording.** If the food packaging has the term "instant" or "flavored" printed on it, stay away! This option is very likely to be ultra-processed.

>> **Opt for packaging with minimal advertising.** Safe, natural foods tend to have minimal advertising. If you see a loud package advertising unrealistic health claims, then chances are this is an ultra-processed item you don't want in your life.

TAKING A CLOSER LOOK AT ULTRA-PROCESSED FOOD

Ultra-processed foods (UPF) are products that are heavily altered from their original form and often contain added sugars, refined starches, unhealthy fats, and additives. UPFs became more processed over time to make them cheaper, last longer, taste better, and be easier to produce and distribute, but these changes often moved foods farther away from their natural and healthier forms. You should review Chapter 5 for a more in-depth analysis detailing both examples and consequences of these bad food choices. While these foods are designed to be convenient and highly palatable, they are linked to weight gain, insulin resistance, heart disease, and other chronic conditions.

Because of these health risks, ultra-processed food has become more than a personal nutrition issue and is now a broader public health concern. Policymakers and health leaders have begun to discuss how the modern food environment makes it harder for people to make healthy choices. This conversation has reached national health agencies and federal leadership, reflecting growing concern about how these foods affect long-term health. Understanding this context helps explain why reducing ultra-processed foods is an important part of weight and metabolic health.

Adequate hydration

Staying hydrated is a simple but often overlooked strategy. Drinking adequate water — about 2.7 liters (91 ounces) for women and 3.7 liters (125 ounces) for men per day — can help manage appetite and support metabolism. Some people confuse thirst with hunger, leading to unnecessary snacking. GLP-RAs may also cause mild nausea, which can be treated with better hydration.

Regular physical activity

Exercise is not mandatory for weight loss with GLP-RAs, but it enhances fat loss, preserves muscle, and improves insulin sensitivity. A combination of cardio (like walking, cycling, or swimming) and strength training (such as bodyweight exercises or lifting weights) is ideal. Aim for at least 150 minutes of moderate aerobic activity per week and include two sessions of resistance training. Even light activity, like taking short walks throughout the day, can make a difference. (See Chapter 5 if you would like to learn more about integrating regular physical activity with your weight-loss medication journey.)

Sleep and stress management

Poor sleep and high stress levels can undermine weight-loss efforts, even while on GLP-RAs. Sleep deprivation alters hunger hormones (ghrelin and leptin), potentially increasing appetite. Aim for seven to nine hours of quality sleep each night. Stress can trigger emotional eating or cravings, especially for high-calorie comfort foods. Stress-reducing practices like meditation, deep breathing, or yoga can improve overall well-being and support consistent weight loss.

Consistent routine and tracking

Building a consistent routine around meals, activity, and sleep can improve adherence to lifestyle changes. Tracking food intake, weight, and physical activity using a journal or an app can increase accountability and identify patterns or obstacles. While GLP-RAs makes weight loss easier for many, behavioral awareness is still key to long-term success. (See Chapter 6 for real-world practices to implement, such as using Apps like MyFitnessPal, Lose It!, Cronometer, and more to aid in your weight-loss journey.)

Defining your success

Remembering that the failure of medication doesn't mean that you failed is important. It means your body didn't respond to one particular approach — and that's valuable information. It helps guide the next steps.

When medication fails, it may be time to reframe what success looks like. Often, the goal of weight loss is tied to a number on the scale, an ideal body size, or even societal expectations. But this framing is narrow — and sometimes counterproductive.

Instead, focus on **health gains**, not just weight loss. Ask yourself these questions:

>> Are my blood sugar and blood pressure under better control?

>> Do I have more energy or better sleep?

>> Is my joint pain less severe?

>> Am I eating more nourishing foods consistently?

>> Am I managing stress more effectively?

Obesity is about more than just weight. This chronic condition is a personification of how your body functions. A person can remain in the "obese" category by BMI standards and still improve their cardiovascular health, insulin sensitivity, liver function, and mental well-being. These improvements matter. They add years to your life. By seeking health gains, you can enrich your life along the weight-loss journey.

In doing so, you can broaden the possibilities of success and create a personal space for sustainable progress that focuses on your mind, body, and soul.

Handling Adverse Reactions and Side Effects

As with any medication, it is important to understand both the benefits and the possible side effects. GLP-RAs can be very effective tools for managing diabetes and obesity, but they work by changing how your body handles digestion, appetite, and blood sugar. Because of this, some side effects are common, especially when starting or adjusting the dose. Knowing what to expect and how to respond can help you use these medications safely and with confidence.

GLP-RAs have become a cornerstone in the management of type 2 diabetes and obesity. Medications such as semaglutide (Ozempic, Wegovy), liraglutide (Victoza, Saxenda), and dulaglutide (Trulicity) are praised for their ability to regulate blood glucose, suppress appetite, slow gastric emptying, and promote significant weight loss (see Chapter 2 if you would like to review are more in-depth discussion of the drugs mechanisms of action of efficacy to assist in losing weight). However, while clinically effective, these agents frequently cause side effects — ranging from mild gastrointestinal discomfort to more serious concerns like pancreatitis or gallbladder disease.

The increasing popularity of GLP-1 medications demands a clear understanding of their side effects and how to manage them. Both healthcare providers and patients must be equipped to recognize adverse events, apply evidence-based interventions, and make adjustments that maintain safety while maximizing benefits. This chapter explores common and rare side effects of GLP-1 RAs, their underlying mechanisms, and strategies for minimizing or managing them.

GLP-1 receptor agonists mimic the action of endogenous GLP-1, an incretin hormone secreted by the gut in response to nutrient ingestion. They act on several physiological systems:

Identifying common side effects

GLP-RA medications work by acting on several organs in the body that help control appetite, blood sugar, and metabolism. Because these same systems are involved in digestion and hormone signaling, they can also be the source of major side effects. This list explains how these organs respond to GLP-RAs and how sometimes that response to medication can mount a negative side effect:

>> **Pancreas:** Stimulates glucose-dependent insulin secretion and inhibits glucagon release

- » **Brain:** Promotes satiety and reduces appetite via hypothalamic pathways
- » **Stomach:** Slows gastric emptying, delaying nutrient absorption reducing postprandial glucose spikes
- » **Cardiovascular system:** Offers benefits such as reduced blood pressure and improved lipid profiles

Despite their advantages, GLP-RAs are associated with a wide range of side effects, primarily due to their impact on the gastrointestinal system and hormone regulation. These sections go through the most common, major side effects and what you can do to manage them.

Nausea

Nausea is the most frequently reported side effect, especially when initiating therapy or increasing dosage. GLP-1 RAs delay gastric emptying and act directly on the central nervous system, where they may trigger nausea centers in the brain. But you can use the following management strategies to minimize the impact:

- » **Follow a slow dose titration.** Start at the lowest dose and increase gradually every 4 weeks (or as recommended).
- » **Eat smaller, low-fat meals.** Fatty foods can worsen nausea.
- » **Avoid lying down after meals.** Helps reduce reflux and indigestion.
- » **Focus on hydration.** Staying hydrated can reduce discomfort.
- » **Use anti-nausea medications.** Short-term use of ondansetron or metoclopramide may be appropriate in some cases.
- » **Wait it out.** Nausea often improves within weeks as the body adjusts.

Vomiting

While less common than nausea, vomiting can occur in susceptible individuals, particularly with higher doses or improper dietary habits. You will find that the side effect of vomiting is caused by a similar effect of GLP-RAs on the gastric emptying. In the case of vomiting, either the capacity of the stomach and the volume in can hold is exceeded, or the central nervous system such as the vagus nerve is overwhelmed leading to vomiting.

You can use the same strategies as for nausea as well as the following:

>> Pause dose escalation: If vomiting is severe, maintain the current dose until symptoms resolve before resuming titration.

>> Assess hydration and electrolytes in cases of prolonged vomiting.

Changes in bowel habits

Both diarrhea and constipation are frequently reported, sometimes alternating in the same patient. GLP-RAs change gut motility (how your gut moves food from the top of your stomach down to the bottom of your colon through the digestion process) and secretions. Some people notice diarrhea, constipation, or a mix of both when taking GLP-RA medications. This happens because these medicines slow down digestion and change how the intestine moves food forward. Slower digestion can lead to constipation, while changes in gut signaling can sometimes cause loose stools. These effects are tied to how the medication works to reduce appetite and calorie intake. While uncomfortable, they are often temporary and related to the same processes that support weight loss.

You can manage changes in bowel habits with these strategies, which differ depending on whether you're experiencing diarrhea or constipation:

>> **For diarrhea:**
  - Stay hydrated with electrolyte solutions. The general recommendation for fluid intake for adults is about 2.7 liters (91 ounces) for women and 3.7 liters (125 ounces) for men per day.
  - Use bulking agents, such as fiber, or over the counter anti-diarrheal medications like loperamide, if needed.
  - Avoid high-fat or spicy foods.

>> **For constipation:**
  - Ensure adequate water intake.
  - Use gentle laxatives (such as polyethylene glycol 3350) short term, using 1 cap-full daily in 8 ounces of water to achieve "apple sauce" consistency of stools.
  - Get physically active to promote bowel regularity.

GETTING LIQUID NUTRITION

There are some FDA-approved formulas on the market which you can purchase to ensure ideal nutrition intake even when you lose your appetite. Many options, such as Kate Farms High Protein, are plant based, lactose free, and gentle on the stomach. This can be especially helpful while your body is adjusting to GLP-RA medications.

Liquid nutrition can help you meet protein and calorie needs without forcing food when eating feels hard. This supports muscle mass, energy, and overall nutrition during weight loss. Using liquid formulas can also reduce nausea by allowing smaller, more frequent intake. These products are not meant to replace all meals long term, but they can be a useful tool to bridge periods of low appetite while you stay on track with your health goals. This means you can achieve the proper nutritional goals while maintaining weight loss and avoiding side effects like nausea thanks to your liquid formula.

Loss of appetite

While losing your appetite is a therapeutic goal for many patients using GLP-RAs for weight loss, excessive appetite suppression can lead to inadequate nutrient intake or malnutrition. But you can manage it by doing the following:

>> Monitor caloric intake, especially protein.

>> Schedule meals so you're eating even without hunger to maintain energy and nutritional adequacy.

>> Take advantage of nutritional counseling to help prevent under-eating or disordered eating behaviors.

Table 8-1 gives you an overview of the most common side effects, the medications they're most common with, and management strategies you may experience when taking various weight-loss medications.

Recognizing severe reactions: When to seek medical help

There are several less common, but very serious potential reactions that your doctor should counsel you about prior to starting GLP-RAs. We recommend always developing a game plan before starting new medications. Your game plan should follow the format:

If *this happens*, then I will recognize, act, and respond by *doing this*.

TABLE 8-1   **Managing Common GLP-RA Side Effects**

Side Effect	Reason	Most Common With	Management Strategies
Nausea	Many GLP-1 receptor agonists slow gastric emptying, leading to feelings of fullness or queasiness.	Semaglutide (Ozempic, Wegovy), liraglutide (Saxenda)	Eat smaller meals, avoid high-fat foods, take medication with food, and titrate dose slowly.
Diarrhea	Medications affecting gut motility or absorption can cause loose stools.	Orlistat, GLP receptor agonists	Increase fiber intake, stay hydrated, monitor diet, and avoid greasy foods.
Constipation	Slower gastric motility from medications like GLP-1 agonists may reduce bowel movement frequency.	Semaglutide, liraglutide	Increase fluid intake, eat high-fiber foods, and use stool softeners if necessary.
Headache	Pain can result from dehydration, low blood sugar, or medication adjustment.	Phentermine-topiramate, naltrexone-bupropion	Ensure adequate hydration, eat regular meals, and monitor blood pressure.
Insomnia	Stimulant medications may increase alertness or disrupt sleep.	Phentermine, phentermine-topiramate	Take medication early in the day, avoid caffeine, and practice good sleep hygiene.
Fatty/oily stools (steatorrhea)	Medications can inhibit fat absorption in the intestines.	Orlistat	Reduce dietary fat intake and be near a restroom after meals.
Dizziness	This is often related to dehydration, low blood pressure, or low blood sugar.	Phentermine, naltrexone-bupropion	Stay hydrated, rise slowly from sitting/lying, and monitor blood glucose.
Increased heart rate	Stimulant effects can activate the sympathetic nervous system.	Phentermine, phentermine-topiramate	Monitor pulse, avoid other stimulants, and report persistent symptoms to provider.
Mood changes (irritability, anxiety)	Some medications affect neurotransmitter levels.	Naltrexone-bupropion	Monitor mental health and report severe symptoms; may need a dose adjustment.

These sections describe what signs and symptoms accompany these reactions to help you recognize them, and we fill in your game plan by offering ways you can respond.

Pancreatitis

Though rare, acute pancreatitis has been reported in patients using GLP-1 medications. Look for these signs and symptoms:

>> Severe abdominal pain radiating to the back

>> Nausea and vomiting

>> Elevated amylase and lipase levels

>> Abnormal findings of pancreas on ultrasound, computed tomography (CT), or magnetic resonance imaging (MRI)

Then manage your reaction with the following actions:

>> Immediate discontinuation of the GLP-1 agent

>> Emergency evaluation and supportive care

WARNING

Do not restart the medication unless another clear cause is found. If pancreatitis occurs while taking a GLP-RA medication, the drug is usually stopped. It should only be restarted if your doctor determines that the pancreatitis was caused by something else, such as gallstones or alcohol use, and not by the medication.

Gallbladder disease

GLP-1 RAs may increase the risk of gallstones or cholecystitis, particularly during rapid weight loss, and monitor for symptoms that occur together, such as:

>> Right upper quadrant pain

>> Jaundice (yellowing of the skin, inside of mouth, or whites of the eyes)

>> Fever

Do the following to monitor and/or prevent a reaction:

>> Ask your doctor to order an ultrasound of the right upper quadrant or gallbladder if symptomatic.

>> Some providers may recommend a special medication called ursodiol in an attempt to prevent this side effect in high-risk patients undergoing rapid weight loss.

Hypoglycemia/low blood sugar

While GLP-1 RAs alone do not typically cause hypoglycemia, the risk increases when combined with insulin or sulfonylureas (for example, Glipizide, Glyburide, or Glimepiride). Recognize hypoglycemia symptoms such as:

>> Pale skin

>> Unexplained fatigue

>> Shaking

>> Sweating

>> Dizziness

>> Irritability or anxiety

>> Blurry vision

>> Loss of consciousness, seizure, or coma

Manage this reaction by doing the following:

>> Adjust co-administered medications (insulin and sulfonylureas) to lower the risk.

>> Encourage regular meals/snacks if needed.

Injection Site Reactions

These are generally mild but may include redness, itching, or nodules. You can manage this by following these strategies:

>> Rotate injection sites regularly.

>> Use proper injection techniques.

>> Consider over the counter topical antihistamines or topical over the counter hydrocortisone if reactions persist.

You can review the more rare, but serious side effects and risks you take with various weight-loss medications in Table 8-2 below. We always recommend discussing with your primary care or specialty provider before changing medications and/or initiating weight-loss medicines. (See Chapter 4 for tips on how you can seek healthcare guidance.)

TABLE 8-2   **Serious Side Effects for GLP-RAs**

Serious Side Effect	Why It Happens	Diagnostics Needed	Treatment	Discontinue Medication?
Pancreatitis	GLP-1 receptor agonists may increase pancreatic enzyme secretion and cause inflammation.	Serum lipase/amylase, abdominal ultrasound or CT scan	Hospitalization, IV fluids, bowel rest, analgesics	Yes, if confirmed
Gallbladder disease (cholelithiasis, cholecystitis)	Rapid weight loss and altered gallbladder motility increase bile stasis and risk of gallstone formation.	Abdominal ultrasound, liver function tests	Pain management, antibiotics if infected, surgical removal if indicated	May require discontinuation depending on severity and recurrence
Severe gastrointestinal obstruction	GLP-1 agonists slow gastric emptying; in rare cases, this may lead to severe obstruction.	Abdominal X-ray, CT scan, endoscopy	Hospitalization, NG tube decompression, possible surgery	Yes, if confirmed
Thyroid C-cell tumors (observed in rodents)	GLP-1 receptors on C-cells may stimulate proliferation (seen in animal studies).	Neck ultrasound, calcitonin levels	Endocrine consultation, surgical evaluation if indicated	Yes, especially if personal or family history of medullary thyroid carcinoma
Acute kidney injury (AKI)	Severe dehydration from nausea/vomiting or decreased oral intake may lead to reduced renal perfusion.	Serum creatinine, BUN, electrolytes, urinalysis	IV hydration, monitoring renal function, supportive care	Temporarily discontinue; may restart with caution after recovery
Hypersensitivity reactions (angioedema, anaphylaxis)	Immune-mediated allergic response to the drug or excipients.	Clinical diagnosis, consider tryptase level, allergy testing	Epinephrine, antihistamines, corticosteroids	Yes, permanently discontinue

Chapter **9**

Applying Alternative Strategies When Medications Don't Work

S ome people expect weight-loss medications to feel like magic, but the truth is that not every medicine works for every person. Sometimes the medication helps at first and then your weight-loss stalls. Sometimes the side effects you experience can get in the way. When this happens, it can feel frustrating, but it does not mean your journey is over. It means you shift your strategy and tap into the many other, unexplored tools that can still work for you. In this chapter, we go deeper into non-medication options that are backed by real research. These tools can support weight loss, improve health, and help maintain your weight-loss momentum even when medication effectiveness hits a wall.

Exploring Non-Pharmacological Options

When medications aren't the whole answer, it helps to look at the bigger picture and explore non-pharmacological options. This means you must consider options that support your body from every angle. There are many effective science-based strategies that do not require medication. Some focus on the food you eat or how you move. Some focus on your mindset. Some focus on your relationship with stress or sleep. These strategies can work on their own, but many people use them alongside medication for maximum effectiveness.

Honing in on holistic care and functional medicine

Holistic care focuses on things like nutrition, sleep, movement, stress, gut health, and emotional well-being. Many people find this approach helps them feel better while slowly losing weight. Functional medicine takes this a step further by looking for root causes like inflammation, hormone imbalance, nutrient deficiencies, or chronic stress. Then your functional medicine physician can help you to create a personalized plan that supports your healing rather than just treating symptoms.

TIP

When you are trying to confirm whether someone is truly trained in functional medicine, there are a few key credentials to look for. The most recognized certification in this field is through the Institute for Functional Medicine, and clinicians who complete their full training hold the title IFM Certified Practitioner or IFMCP. Some clinicians also complete coursework with the American Academy of Anti-Aging Medicine, which uses the credential FAAMFM or FAARM, although this pathway is broader and not specific to functional medicine alone.

Dietary enhancement

When medication does not give your desired results, adjusting your nutrition can help. These changes do not have to be extreme. They can be small steps that support steady progress. Focus on adjusting in the following ways:

» **Protein:** One key strategy is focusing on protein. Research shows that higher protein intake supports satiety and protects muscle during weight loss. Many people feel best with 25 to 30 percent of calories from protein, but you do not have to count every gram. You can simply build most meals around a protein source like chicken, turkey, fish, tofu, beans, eggs, or Greek yogurt.

» **Mediterranean diet:** The Mediterranean diet is an eating pattern built around vegetables, fruits, whole grains, beans, nuts, olive oil, and lean proteins like fish and poultry, with minimal processed foods and sweets. The Mediterranean diet has some of the strongest evidence for steady and sustainable weight loss, and it is not even built around strict calorie limits. In one large study, people who followed this style of eating lost between 4.4 and 10.1 kilograms over a year.

>> **Sugar:** Sugar may not always be the enemy. A recent year-long study compared adults following a healthy low-sugar diet either with or without the use of non-sugar sweeteners. People using sweeteners maintained an extra 1.6 kg of weight loss and showed healthier gut microbiota, especially more SCFA-producing species. Importantly, no metabolic harm was detected in glucose, cholesterol, or heart markers. The only difference between groups was replacement of sugary foods with sweetener-based alternatives, while total added sugar remained less than 10 percent for both. The study challenges the WHO's 2023 guidance advising against sweeteners and suggests context matters.

>> **Fiber:** You should consider increasing fiber. Fiber supplements can make your weight-loss journey easier because fiber helps you feel full sooner and stay full longer. In one study, people who used a higher-fiber, higher-protein shake before meals lost 3.3 kilograms in 12 weeks, compared with 1.8 kilograms in the lower-fiber group. Fiber slows digestion, increases the thickness of food in the stomach, and supports gut bacteria. This can help control your blood sugar and your appetite signals. Most healthy adults are advised to aim for 20 to 35 grams of fiber per day, or about 10 to 13 grams per 1,000 calories eaten.

TIP

If you want help with meal ideas, websites like Skinnytaste, Budget Bytes, Diet Doctor, and the American Heart Association Healthy Recipes page offer free meal plans built around balanced nutrition.

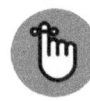

REMEMBER

GLP-RAs reduce appetite and slow gastric emptying, which naturally helps users feel full with less food. This effect can be optimized by practicing mindful eating where you pay attention to hunger cues, eat slowly, and avoid distractions, like phones or screens, during meals. Eating more slowly gives GLP-RAs time to work and helps prevent overeating. Portion control is also important, even if you're feeling less hungry.

Lifestyle modifications

Effective lifestyle management for weight loss starts with creating a consistent calorie deficit through balanced, nutrient-dense meals that emphasize vegetables, lean proteins, whole grains, and high-fiber foods, which have been shown to improve satiety and metabolic health. Regular physical activity is equally important, and guidelines recommend at least 150 minutes per week of moderate aerobic exercise plus two days of resistance training to preserve muscle mass during weight loss.

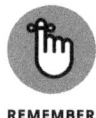

Evidence from the Diabetes Prevention Program demonstrates that even modest weight loss of 5 to 7 percent achieved through diet and physical activity can significantly reduce the risk of developing diabetes.

To set yourself up for success incorporate these strategies:

>> **Tracking food intake, physical activity, and daily habits** — whether through journals or digital tools — helps improve awareness and accountability, which research shows can double the likelihood of success.

>> **Behavioral strategies** such as setting realistic goals, planning meals in advance, and reducing environmental triggers like highly processed snack foods support long-term adherence.

>> **Get adequate sleep and manage stress** because they play key roles. Poor sleep and chronic stress increase hunger hormones and cravings.

>> **Social support,** whether from family, peers, or structured programs, has been linked to better adherence and sustained weight loss.

Because combining dietary improvements, increased physical activity, consistent self-monitoring, and behavioral support creates the strongest evidence-based foundation for effective and lasting weight loss, we cover all of these lifestyle adjustments in the following sections.

Physical fitness

A major study involving nearly 400,000 adults found that cardiorespiratory fitness (CRF) predicts longevity more strongly than body weight. Fit individuals who are overweight or obese had no significant increase in mortality risk compared with fit people of normal weight. In contrast, unfit individuals regardless of BMI had a two to three times higher risk of death. Physical fitness is a separate goal that can be achieved at the same time as weight loss which you should consider. This fact highlights the importance of getting your body moving with cardio, strength, and high-intensity exercises. If you are seeking specific guidance on exercises which will best support your weight loss while on GLP-RAs, then refer back to Chapter 5.

Because all age groups have different needs, consider these goals to see how simple a workout plan can be:

>> **Children (6 to 12 years old)** should be focused on building fun movement habits, improving motor skills, and reducing sedentary time. Aim for 30 to 45 minutes of a mix of cardio, such as jumping rope or biking, strength

training, and engaging agility like hopscotch or obstacle courses. Cooling down can be simple stretching or children's yoga.

>> **Teens (13 to 18 years old)** should focus on building aerobic endurance and learning proper strength-training form. Aim for 45 to 60 minutes that includes moderate cardio like brisk walking, running, or cycling, along with full-body strength exercises such as squats, lunges, push-ups, and core work. This age is ideal for developing confidence, consistency, and healthy exercise habits.

>> **Adults (19 to 29 years old)** should work on improving cardiovascular fitness and starting structured strength training. Aim for 45 to 60 minutes with a balance of moderate to vigorous cardio and full-body resistance training. This helps build muscle, support metabolism, and establish long-term routines.

>> **Adults (30 to 65 years old)** should combine low impact cardio with resistance training to preserve muscle and joint health. Aim for 40 to 50 minutes that includes steady cardio like walking, cycling, or swimming, plus strength exercises for major muscle groups and some balance work. This approach supports metabolic health and reduces injury risk.

>> **Adults (over 65 years old)** should focus on maintaining muscle, improving balance, and reducing fall risk. Aim for 30 to 40 minutes of low impact activity that includes strength exercises like chair squats and wall push-ups, balance activities, and gentle cardio such as walking or water aerobics. The goal is to support independence and daily function.

Hydration

Staying hydrated is a simple but often overlooked strategy. You must ensure that you are drinking adequate water, typically around 8 to 10 cups per day, to help manage appetite and support metabolism.

TIP

Some people confuse thirst with hunger, leading to unnecessary snacking. When you get a hunger craving, try drinking 8 ounces of water, first. GLP-RAs may also cause mild nausea, which can be lessened by adequate hydration (see Chapter 8 for more on side effects).

Sleep and stress management

Poor sleep and high stress levels can undermine weight-loss efforts, even while on GLP-RAs. Sleep deprivation alters hunger hormones (ghrelin and leptin), potentially increasing appetite. Aim for the right amount of sleep by following these guidelines:

>> **Children 6 to 12 years:** Nine to twelve hours per night

>> **Teenagers 13 to 18 years:** Eight to ten hours per night

>> **Adults (all ages):** Seven to nine hours per night

Stress can trigger emotional eating or cravings, especially for high-calorie comfort foods. Stress-reducing practices like meditation, deep breathing, or yoga can improve overall well-being and support consistent weight loss.

Consistent routine and tracking

Building a consistent routine around meals, activity, and sleep can improve adherence to lifestyle changes. Tracking your food intake, weight, and physical activity using a journal or an app can increase accountability and identify patterns or obstacles. While GLP-RAs makes weight loss easier for many, behavioral awareness is still key to your long-term success.

Behavioral Therapy and Support Groups

Behavioral therapy is one of the strongest tools for weight management when medication alone is not enough. The goal is not to change who you are. The goal is to strengthen the habits and thoughts that support health. Cognitive behavioral therapy, motivational interviewing, and acceptance and commitment therapy help people develop consistent routines, manage emotional eating, and handle setbacks without quitting. You have a lot of options to choose from:

>> **Licensed therapists** trained in weight management can be found through Psychology Today, the Obesity Medicine Association, or insurance directories. Weight management programs boast a 5 to 15 percent total body weight loss at one year.

Many therapists now offer telehealth, which makes sessions easier to fit into a busy schedule. And some people benefit from short-term structured programs that focus specifically on eating behavior.

>> **Group-based programs** like Weight Watchers, TOPS (Take Off Pounds Sensibly), and the National Diabetes Prevention Program (DPP) are also backed by strong evidence. Research shows that DPP participants lose 5 to 7 percent of their weight on average and reduce their risk of diabetes. You can find a local DPP program through the CDC website. Many programs meet online and offer coaching, meal ideas, and weekly check-ins.

Of these weight management groups, one stands out due to active patient engagement: Accomplish Health. This team claims substantially better results, including greater than 20 percent average weight loss at 12 months and 80 percent of patients achieving at least or greater than 10 percent TBWL.

>> **Online platforms** like AbleTo, BetterHelp, and Talkspace can connect people with therapists who specialize in weight, stress, and behavior change.

>> **Support groups** are another useful option. People often feel less alone when they connect with others who understand their struggles. The Obesity Action Coalition provides you with free online community groups. Programs like Overeaters Anonymous and SMART Recovery help when you feel stuck in cycles of emotional or binge eating. These groups are not about shame. They are about providing you with support, perspective, and accountability.

Integrative and Complementary Approaches

Some people like to explore integrative options along with standard weight-loss strategies. You may find that these approaches help your sleep, stress, digestion, and inflammation, all areas that can affect your weight.

Try these integrative approaches:

>> **You can try mind-body practices like yoga, Pilates, or tai chi.** These activities lower stress hormones and improve how your body moves. They also help you notice hunger and fullness. You can find free beginner classes on YouTube, DoYogaWithMe, and the Peloton app.

>> **You may also want to try acupuncture for stress or appetite support.** Results are different for everyone, but some people sleep better and feel calmer after treatment. You can search for licensed providers through the National Certification Commission for Acupuncture and Oriental Medicine.

>> **Try foods that impact your gut health.** Some people notice easier digestion or better appetite control with probiotics or fermented foods. Trusted websites like Cleveland Clinic, Harvard Health, and Johns Hopkins offer simple guidance on this topic.

>> **Massage therapy** is another option for stress and sleep support. You can schedule services through Massage Envy, Zeel, or Soothe.

TIP

Many people get the best results when they combine several integrative tools. You may find that gentle movement, simple nutrition changes, therapy, and stress support work together when medication alone is not enough.

Steering Clear of the Hype

Some options sound great in theory, but they really don't work. So people trying hard to lose weight end up disappointed by the results. To help you avoid taking part in programs, systems, and new-fangled products that offer no real weight-loss benefit, we break down the alternatives here that aren't worth your time or money.

Peptides

There is a growing cultural enthusiasm around peptides that is not supported by strong scientific evidence. Most peptides are promoted for wellness, anti-aging, fat loss, or rejuvenation. These products largely lack valid human research trials. Many claims originate from rodent studies or commercial marketing rather than clinical science.

WARNING

Off-label peptide use is spreading despite minimal safety data, creating a landscape driven more by hype than evidence. The current lineup of peptide products includes compounds like BPC-157, CJC-1295, Ipamorelin, Tesamorelin, MOTS-c, and AOD-9604.

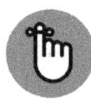

REMEMBER

The peptide boom is mostly speculation wrapped in marketing, not a validated medical revolution. BPC-157, CJC-1295, Ipamorelin, MOTS-c, AOD-9604, are technically illegal to sell for human use in the U.S. Among those clinics willing to dispense these items, quality control is a major issue. Growth hormone–related peptides such as CJC-1295 and Ipamorelin may increase growth hormone levels, but studies have not shown actual fat loss or BMI reduction. AOD-9604 has a few small human studies suggesting tiny changes in fat measurements, but no real reductions in body weight. MOTS-c has only one small pilot study showing slight metabolic changes but no measurable weight loss. Tesamorelin is the only FDA-approved peptide on this list, and even then, it's approved only for HIV-associated lipodystrophy. This peptide has shown reductions in visceral fat but does not produce significant overall weight loss. In sum, these peptides typically produce 0 to 2 percent total body weight loss (TBWL) at best, far below what is needed for metabolic improvement.

Hyperbaric oxygen therapy (HBOT)

Traditionally used medically for wound healing and decompression sickness, hyperbaric oxygen therapy (HBOT) has only been studied in very small human pilot studies for its potential to facilitate weight loss. Across these small trials, the reported weight changes are not clinically meaningful, typically well under 1 to 2 percent total body weight loss. Evidence is extremely limited, with other small pilot studies suggesting minor changes in inflammation or metabolic markers. This is not going to be a stand-alone solution for you.

Red-light therapy

Red-light therapy (photobiomodulation) has been theorized to help with your weight loss by boosting your cellular activity and increasing energy use in fat cells, but human studies are very small. You may see a small drop in measurements like one to three centimeters in abdominal circumference. This is mostly fluid loss and not real fat loss. Weight change is usually 0 to 1 percent total body weight. This amount does not improve health, and the effect fades once you stop the treatments. It works more like cosmetic contouring than true weight loss. So, while this option may help boost your confidence, it is unlikely to have a dramatic effect on your weight.

Cryotherapy

Cryotherapy is theorized to help your weight loss by making the body burn more calories when it gets very cold, but human studies are very small. The cold exposure creates a short burst of extra calorie burn. This increase is small and does not lead to real weight loss. Most studies show 0 to 1 percent total body weight loss (TBWL). Many show no weight change at all. The effect on your body does not last once the session ends.

"Fat-burning" injections

Fat-burning injections are supposed to help with your weight loss by boosting your metabolism and improving how your body uses fat. There are no good human studies that test these injections by themselves. Most people who get them are also dieting. Any weight loss usually comes from eating fewer calories and not from the injectable medicine. When weight change is reported, it is 0 to 1 percent total body weight. These injections are popular in medical spas, and so you may see them offered as spa treatments. They can also contain vitamins and amino acids. There is no solid evidence that they cause real fat loss. The benefits you see usually come from the diet plan you have already selected at the same time.

Detoxes, cleanses, and fast-mimicking kits

Detoxes and cleanse kits claim to help with weight loss by flushing out toxins and giving the digestive system a break. They mostly lead to water loss and a short-term, very low caloric intake. You may see the scale drop by one to three percent, but this is not real fat loss. True fat loss through these methods is zero percent. The weight you do lose almost always comes back once normal eating starts again. These programs can also feel hard to follow and are not meant for long-term use.

Spot-fat treatments

Spot-fat treatments, whether through ultrasound cavitation, radiofrequency heat, or laser lipo, are theorized to shrink fat in one specific area of your body by using heat, sound waves, or light. However, human studies are small. These treatments can reduce measurements by one to three centimeters in your treated area. This change is temporary and does not affect your total body weight. Total body weight loss stays at zero percent. They do not improve metabolism or overall health, and they are used mainly in cosmetic clinics, not in medical weight-loss programs.

Brown fat "activation" devices

Brown fat activation devices are suggested to help with weight loss by turning your brown fat on. Your activated brown fat can burn calories to create heat. Human studies are very small and mostly look at temperature changes, not real weight loss. None of these popular devices, commonly sold online, are FDA-approved for weight loss. The amount of brown fat they activate is far too small to change body weight. Total body weight loss stays at zero percent in studies, and there is no sustained fat loss at all. These tools remain more of a theory than a proven weight-loss method.

Chapter **10**

Exploring Weight-Loss Surgery

I f you've tried weight-loss medications like GLP-1 agonists and incorporated lifestyle management changes but haven't seen the results you hoped for, bariatric surgery can open a new door of weight-loss possibilities for you. These procedures work in ways that go beyond medication, helping to change how your body handles hunger, fullness, and metabolism and even restore a normal glucose set point. Many people experience significant and lasting weight loss, along with improvements in conditions like diabetes, high blood pressure, and sleep apnea. Surgery can also make it easier for you to maintain healthy habits by giving you a "reset" both physically and mentally. While it's a big step that requires consideration and commitment, it can be a life-changing tool to help you reach goals that felt out of reach before. With the right support team, bariatric surgery can be a powerful partner on your journey to better health and quality of life.

TIP

Bariatric surgery may present an opportunity for you to optimize your health prior to other specialty surgery, such as joint arthroplasty, abdominal wall hernia repair, or organ transplantation. Before your bariatric surgery, you'll work with a supportive team of experts who are here to help you get in the best shape possible. The goal is to position you and your body for a safe follow on surgery and smooth recovery. Together, you'll focus on changes that can lower your risks and set you up for success. Your surgeon will guide you on when the time is right for your procedure. Remember, severe obesity is a long-term condition, and surgery is just one step in your journey. Even after your first bariatric surgery, you may benefit from other treatments or follow-up procedures to help you achieve and maintain your goals.

To help you navigate through the process, from making the decision to what to do after surgery, we cover all of the topics you need to know in this chapter as well as help you understand what to expect from the process and what to discuss with your care team.

Determining Eligibility Criteria with Pre-Surgery Assessments

The 2022 American Society of Metabolic and Bariatric Surgery (ASMBS) and International Federation for the Surgery of Obesity and Metabolic Disorders (IFSO) guideline provides patients with major bariatric surgery updates. In contrast to the original 1991 literature, this new guideline commits to several new, bold statements.

In the past, people with a BMI over 35 could only get surgery if they already had a serious health issue caused by obesity (like diabetes, sleep apnea, or severe joint pain). The new guideline makes it easier so you don't need to wait until your health gets worse before surgery is an option.

You may be a candidate for weight-loss (bariatric) surgery if:

>> Your BMI is 35 or higher, even if you don't have other health problems.

>> Your BMI is lower than 35 but you also have conditions like diabetes or high blood pressure. The guideline specifically states that bariatric surgery should be considered if you have type 2 diabetes and BMI greater than 30.

>> You have tried medications like GLP-1s but haven't been able to lose enough weight and still have a BMI 30 to 34.9.

Understanding why BMI alone does not tell your full story

This section highlights why obesity care cannot focus on the number on the scale alone. Conditions like obesity with impaired mobility show how excess weight can limit function, independence, and daily life in ways that numbers do not capture.

Obesity is a chronic inflammatory condition, and care should be personalized to help people regain function and meet them where they are. As a patient, you should expect and demand this more human, function-focused approach to your care.

Obesity with impaired mobility (OBOMOB) means that extra weight makes it hard to walk without help, often requiring devices like a cane, walker, or scooter, and it carries health risks beyond weight alone. Patients who meet the OBOMOB criteria should be considered for bariatric surgery. Core requirements are that patients have a BMI equal to or great than 30 and demonstrate clinically significant impairment in independent ambulation directly attributable to excess body weight. Plus one of the following must be true:

>> **Dependence on mobility device** (walker, rollator, cane, scooter, or electric wheelchair) for routine ambulation beyond short distances (great than 10 meters).

>> **Marked gait limitation** documented by provider inability to ambulate without assistance, frequent rests due to weight-related pain or dyspnea).

>> **Physical performance testing** (such as a timed up-and-go, 6-minute walk test) showing clinically significant limitation attributed primarily to obesity-related biomechanical or musculoskeletal strain.

REMEMBER

OBOMOB is not defined by weight or body mass index (BMI) alone. Instead, it focuses on how extra weight affects a person's ability to move around. This diagnosis is made when someone has noticeable difficulty walking on their own because their weight places extra strain on their joints, muscles, or overall movement. A key part of OBOMOB is whether a person needs to rely on a mobility aid, such as a cane, walker, rollator, scooter, or powered wheelchair. The goal is to better describe patients who have obesity and physical limitations that may prevent normal lifestyle interventions, impede the ability to take medications, and who may need step-up therapies. This condition is important to recognize because people with OBOMOB may face higher risks of health problems like blood pooling in the legs, loss of physical fitness, falls, or social isolation, which aren't always reflected by BMI numbers alone.

Considering age when thinking about surgery

The ASMBS says there's no strict age cutoff for bariatric surgery, meaning even older adults can be candidates if they're healthy enough for the procedure. For example, if a 72-year-old with obesity and type 2 diabetes hasn't had success losing weight on tirzepatide, surgery may still be an option if their overall health and mobility are good and the potential benefits outweigh the risks.

TIP

Children and adolescents with either a BMI greater than 120 percent of the 95th percentile and a major co-morbidity, or a BMI greater than 140 percent of the 95th percentile, should be considered for bariatric surgery. To understand these criteria better, consider this example: A 14-year-old's 95th percentile BMI is 25. If their BMI is over 30 (which equals 120 percent of 25) *and* they have severe sleep apnea, they might be a candidate. If their BMI is over 35 (which is 140 percent of 25), they could be considered even without another major health problem.

This 2022 bariatric surgery statement can come as an aggressive shock to many parents. However, the rising obesity epidemic is because obesity is a multifactorial syndrome. If your child cannot significantly alter their obesity path with lifestyle options and medications, then bariatric surgery is a proper, safe, evidence-based option. This can help to prevent or treat significant complications such as type 2 diabetes or fatty liver.

TECHNICAL
STUFF

Previously called non-alcoholic fatty liver disease (NAFLD), "fatty liver" is now termed metabolic dysfunction–associated steatotic liver disease (MASLD).

This consideration for bariatric surgery should only ever occur for your child after evaluation by a multidisciplinary team in an obesity specialty center. This bariatric surgery recommendation by ASBMS parallels the 2023 recommendation from the American Academy of Pediatrics (AAP) clinical practice guideline for evaluating and treating children with obesity. The AAP guideline specifically states that bariatric surgery may be offered to adolescents aged 13 years and older who have severe obesity.

Considering Pre-Surgery Assessment and Preparation

Preparing for surgery is more than just the days and weeks leading up to it. You also have to consider how you'll prepare yourself to return home and recover. These sections take the guesswork out of it all and let you know what to expect.

Understanding the assessment checklist

Before your bariatric surgery, you'll have a thorough assessment to make sure the procedure is safe and right for you. Here is an example checklist that you can use with your team. This modified checklist follows a familiar design that your bariatric medicine team may give to you. (Many of these are the same lab tests described in deeper detail in Chapter 6.)

Your team will conduct:

>> A comprehensive physical assessment, including medical history

>> Laboratory testing, including routine labs like fasting blood glucose and lipid panel as well as nutrient screening

>> Cardiovascular and sleep assessments

>> Thyroid and endocrine evaluation

>> Gastrointestinal and liver evaluation

TECHNICAL STUFF

The American Association for the Study of Liver Diseases (AASLD) 2023 guidance does not recommend universal screening for metabolic dysfunction–associated steatotic liver disease (MASLD) in the general population. Instead, your team should consider targeted screening for you if you're at higher risk and have type 2 diabetes.

>> Possible imaging, such as abdominal ultrasound, based on your team's recommendations

>> Lifestyle and medicine evaluation

>> Evaluate nutrition and behavioral health

>> Discuss risk reduction and counseling for needs like contraception guidance and smoking cessation

Preparing for easier recovery from surgery

Enhanced Recovery After Bariatric Surgery (ERABS) is a plan designed by ASBMS to help you heal faster, feel better, and get home sooner after weight-loss surgery. Instead of just focusing on the operation itself, ERABS looks at your whole journey: before, during, and after surgery. Part of this plan includes breathing exercises you can do daily before your surgery to help you expand the lungs, prevent pneumonia, and improve oxygenation, all of which help you when healing and recovering from surgery. Deep breathing can be practiced by slowly inhaling through the nose, holding for 3 to 5 seconds, exhaling fully, and repeating for ten breaths every hour while awake. Alternatively, you can try incentive spirometry. Incentive spirometry involves using a handheld device to take slow, deep breaths, aiming to keep the indicator at your target level for ten breaths each session, eight to ten times a day.

In addition to your breathing exercises, your best chance of a great surgical outcome includes performing regular, pre-surgery leg exercises. You can do simple leg exercises such as ankle pumps, heel raises, and marching in place. These exercises can boost your heart to leg blood flow and lower your risk of blood clots after surgery. You should aim to perform these for five to ten minutes every one to two hours while awake, maintaining a gentle pace that keeps your heart rate in a comfortable conversational zone — usually around 50 to 70 percent of your maximum heart rate (which is roughly 220 minus your age).

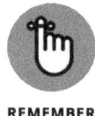

REMEMBER

Follow pre-op nutrition instructions, including clear carbohydrate-containing liquids up to two hours before surgery, and follow any other instructions given to you by your medical team, including taking any prescriptions, reading through instructions you're given.

Deciding whether to continue your GLP-RA medication

REMEMBER

The ASMBS, in collaboration with other medical societies, recommends that you continue taking your GLP-RA medications in the lead-up to elective surgery, including bariatric surgical procedures.

However, if you are at high risk of gastrointestinal (GI) side effects — such as nausea, vomiting, bloating, or delayed stomach emptying, you may need to commit to a liquid-only diet for 24 hours before surgery. You should notify your bariatric surgery team beforehand because adjustments to the anesthesia plan may be considered to reduce the risk of aspiration (food content from the stomach are vomiting directly into your lungs).

This approach emphasizes a shared decision-making model, where the surgical team, anesthesiologists, and prescribing clinicians collaborate to weigh the continued metabolic benefits of GLP RA therapy against your personal risks. In rare cases, a procedure may even be delayed if your GI risk remains unacceptably high.

Recognizing Types of Weight-Loss Surgery

The most common bariatric surgeries you may encounter include Roux-en-Y Gastric Bypass (RYGB), Sleeve Gastrectomy (SG), and more advanced options like Biliopancreatic Diversion with Duodenal Switch (BPD/DS) and Single Anastomosis Duodeno-Ileal Bypass with Sleeve (SADI-S).

RYGB and SG are the most frequently performed, with RYGB offering you the possibility of both weight loss and metabolic benefits, especially if you suffer from diabetes and/or reflux. SG may provide you with a simpler, tried-and-true approach with good results and fewer anatomical changes.

BPD/DS and SADI-S can each deliver you the most powerful weight loss and diabetes remission options, particularly if you have a very high BMI or severe metabolic disease. You must consider these with caution because BPD/DS and SADI-S both require the most intensive lifelong vitamin supplementation and follow-up care.

We cover all these options in the following sections so you understand what they are and how they can impact your weight-loss efforts.

Roux-en-Y Gastric Bypass (RYGB)

Considered the gold standard for many years, RYGB delivers substantial weight loss (about 26 percent total body weight loss) and excellent improvement in obesity-related conditions, especially acid reflux and type 2 diabetes. This surgery makes your stomach smaller and reroutes your intestines so you absorb fewer calories. Your post operative risks include development dumping syndrome, marginal ulcers, and internal hernias, and it requires lifelong supplements. It's a strong choice for many patients with good long-term data.

TIP

This option may be best for patients with diabetes, acid reflux, or those wanting a well-studied, balanced option for weight loss and health improvement.

Sleeve Gastrectomy (SG)

Currently the most frequently performed bariatric surgery worldwide, SG is technically simpler with fewer immediate complications and good weight loss (about 22 percent total body weight loss). This surgery removes about 80 percent of your stomach, leaving a narrow "sleeve" that helps you feel full faster and reduces hunger hormones. However, it can cause or worsen your acid reflux. Some studies indicate that you may achieve less weight loss over the long term compared to bypass or malabsorptive procedures. It's best if you are a lower-risk patient or if you are not ready for more complex surgeries discussed below.

TIP

This option may be best for patients who want simpler, shorter surgery with good weight loss and no intestinal rerouting.

Biliopancreatic Diversion with Duodenal Switch (BPD/DS)

This surgery has the highest average weight loss (about 35 to 40 percent) and best remission rates for type 2 diabetes, but it's also the most complex. This operation combines a sleeve stomach with a major rerouting of your intestines. BPD/DS also carries the highest risk for you to develop long-term vitamin and nutrient deficiencies. The downside is that BPD/DS creates a higher risk for you to develop long-term nutritional deficiencies and diarrhea/steatorrhea, requiring strict life-long vitamin supplementation and frequent lab monitoring. It's generally best for patients with severe obesity who can commit to rigorous follow-up.

TIP

This option may be best for patients with very high BMI or severe metabolic disease who can commit to intensive follow-up and supplementation.

Single Anastomosis Duodeno-Ileal Bypass with Sleeve (SADI-S)

SADI-offers results nearly as good as BPD/DS (about 30 to 39 percent total body weight loss). This surgery is like the DS but with one intestinal connection instead of two, making the surgery a bit simpler. As a slightly simpler anatomic restricting, SADI-S also confers fewer surgical risks than BPD/DS. SADI-S still requires your rigorous commitment to vitamin supplementation and monitoring for digestive side effects. SADI-S is growing in popularity as a balance between effectiveness and complexity.

TIP

This option may be best for patients who are committed to long-term follow-up and want stronger weight loss than sleeve or bypass with slightly fewer surgical steps than DS.

TIP

While you may see information on the web describing either the Adjustable Gastric Banding or Vertical Banded Gastroplasty (Stomach Stapling), neither of these bariatric surgical approaches are commonly performed today due to lower long-term success and higher revision rates.

Examining the Surgery Process: What to Expect Before and After

For bariatric surgery, you'll usually arrive at the hospital in the morning of your procedure. You will get checked in by the surgical team. You'll be given anesthesia so you're asleep and pain-free while the surgeon operates. Typically, the operation involves the surgeon cutting small "keyhole" incisions into your body so that a tiny camera can be inserted to guide the work. This is called laparoscopy. The surgery itself can take one to four hours depending on the type you and your team agreed on. Afterward you'll wake up in the recovery area where nurses monitor your breathing, pain, and vital signs. Most people stay in the hospital one to three days, start on a clear liquid diet, and are given instructions for gradually reintroducing foods while resting and walking to aid healing.

After your surgery, you'll need to:

>> Attend follow-up visits as scheduled.

>> Follow nutrition and supplement guidance, typically with a registered dietician.

>> Resume physical activity.

>> Participate in support groups or online communities.

>> Keep a food/activity log or use an app for tracking.

>> Keep up your routine, medical monitoring, and prescribed medications.

>> Report persistent diarrhea, constipation, or oily stools as well as new or worsening reflux.

>> Watch for complications.

WARNING

Contact your provider immediately if you have:

>> Persistent nausea, vomiting, or abdominal pain.

>> Rapid heart rate, fever, or difficulty breathing.

>> Signs of dehydration or inability to tolerate fluids.

>> Unexplained hypoglycemia (shakiness, confusion, sweating).

>> Persistent reflux or regurgitation.

Screening and lab tests are important to your overall health, recovery, and maintenance. So your doctor should schedule you for several different labs and screenings after surgery. Your doctor will discuss your need for and the timing of the following with you:

>> Complete blood count (CBC)

>> Comprehensive metabolic panel (CMP)

>> Iron studies (ferritin, iron, TIBC)

- » Vitamin B12 and folate

- » Vitamin D (25-OH) and calcium

- » Thiamine (B1)

- » Fat-soluble vitamins (A, E, K)

- » Zinc and copper

- » HbA1c

- » Lipid panel

- » Bone density (DEXA scan)

- » Endoscopy

- » Abdominal imaging

Altering Your Diet after Surgery

After bariatric surgery, your diet changes in stages to allow your stomach and digestive system to heal, prevent complications, and support long–term weight loss. Here's a clear breakdown based on ASMBS guidelines and common surgical program recommendations:

- » **Stage 1: Clear liquids (days 1 and 2)**

  - Start right after surgery, usually in the hospital.

  - Sip slowly on water, sugar-free clear broths, decaf tea, or sugar-free gelatin.

  - Avoid carbonation, caffeine, and sugar with the goal of staying hydrated.

- » **Stage 2: Full liquids (days 3 to 14)**

  - Add protein shakes, low-fat milk, strained soups, and sugar-free yogurt.

  - Aim for 60 to 80 grams of protein/day and 48 to 64 oz fluids daily.

  - Drink slowly, no straws, and no drinking with meals.

- » **Stage 3: Pureed foods (weeks 3 to 4)**

  - Eat soft, smooth foods like mashed beans, blended lean meats, scrambled eggs, pureed vegetables, and soft fruits.

  - Keep protein the priority and limit fats and added sugars.

> **Stage 4: Soft foods (weeks 5 to 6)**

- Progress to soft, tender foods you can mash with a fork — fish, ground turkey, cooked vegetables, peeled fruits.

- Chew thoroughly and eat slowly to avoid discomfort.

> **Stage 5: Regular bariatric diet (after 6-plus weeks)**

- Focus on protein first at each meal (lean meats, fish, eggs, dairy, legumes), followed by non-starchy vegetables and then small amounts of fruit or whole grains.

- Avoid high-sugar, high-fat foods, and carbonated beverages.

- Lifelong vitamin/mineral supplements are required based on your surgery type.

REMEMBER

Follow these key lifelong rules for eating after you recover from surgery:

> Eat small, slow meals and chew thoroughly.

> Avoid drinking fluids 30 minutes before and after meals.

> Make protein your main meal focus, followed by vegetables.

> Take your bariatric vitamins and minerals every day.

Exploring Alternatives When Surgery Is Not Right for You

For some people, non surgical weight-loss procedures may be a better fit than bariatric surgery. These approaches can offer you meaningful results with lower risks and quicker recovery. Some of your options potentially include:

> **Endoscopic Sleeve Gastroplasty (ESG)** shrinks the stomach using sutures placed through a scope, helping you feel full sooner without cutting or rerouting the intestines. Conversely, you may prefer the Intragastric balloons which are placed by a gastroenterologist endoscopically to temporarily occupy space in your stomach to decrease appetite and support portion control.

> **Duodenal Mucosal Resurfacing (DMR)** uses heat or other methods to "reset" the first part of the small intestine through precise tissue injury. You can think of this sort of like acupuncture with an endoscope. DMR could help

you to improve blood sugar control and possibly aid you in achieving weight loss, especially if you have type 2 diabetes.

>> **Gastric Botox** injects botulin toxin into the lining and muscles of your stomach by a gastroenterologist using an endoscope to relax your stomach muscles to slow emptying. This may help you feel fuller longer, though its effects are temporary (usually lasting six to twelve weeks).

These approaches can be ideal for patients who are not ready for surgery, have lower BMI, want less downtime, or need a bridge to future bariatric surgery while still making progress toward their health goals.

TECHNICAL
STUFF

A recent analysis compared semaglutide to Endoscopic Sleeve Gastroplasty (ESG) using cost-effectiveness modeling. For semaglutide to match ESG's value, it would need to cost $24 to $150 per month, far below its current U.S. price of $500 to $670 per month. At prices above $300 per month, semaglutide becomes less cost-effective than ESG. New modeling shows ESG provides more weight loss, better quality-adjusted life-years (QALYs), and lower total costs over five years. The implication is that semaglutide's high price remains a barrier to being competitive against procedural treatments. With the advent of the "TrumpRx" deal to drive down costs, this paradigm may soon shift. See Chapter 4 for more information about cost.

4

The Part of Tens

Check out the ten most effective medications ranked with clear explanations.

Look through the highlights of ten essential studies that can guide your decisions.

Consider ten non-medication strategies that still deliver meaningful results.

Chapter **11**

Top Ten Weight-Loss Medications Ranked by Effectiveness

The top ten weight-loss medicines each have their own mix of strengths and drawbacks and understanding them can help you make a choice that works for your health and lifestyle. Some options are pills, others are injections, and their effectiveness, tolerability, and convenience can differ greatly, so weighing these factors with your healthcare team is key.

On the pro side, many — like tirzepatide and semaglutide — deliver double-digit percentage weight loss and can also improve conditions such as type 2 diabetes, blood pressure, and cholesterol. On the con side, most require ongoing use to maintain results, can have side effects like nausea or GI discomfort (see Chapter 8 for more on dealing with side effects), and vary in cost and insurance coverage.

We cover the basics of these top medications in this chapter so you can quickly see their effectiveness, side effects, and more. Knowing these rankings can help you and your healthcare team choose a treatment that matches your goals, medical history, and lifestyle so you have the best chance at safe, lasting results. (See Chapter 2 for more in-depth information about each medication.)

Tirzepatide (Mounjaro, Zepbound)

If you're looking at the most effective weight-loss medicines available today, the top two winners on the list are derived from tirzepatide (Mounjaro, Zepbound), which in clinical trials has helped people lose an average of 20 to 22 percent of their total body weight over about seventy-two weeks.

Reference: Jastreboff AM, et al. Tirzepatide Once Weekly for the Treatment of Obesity. *N Engl J Med.* 2022;387:205-216. doi:10.1056/NEJMoa2206038

From a cost perspective, tirzepatide is also one of the most expensive options. The list price typically ranges from about $1,080 to $1,300 per month for name-brand versions. Some self-pay or manufacturer assistance programs may lower the monthly cost to around $499 for select doses, but access and eligibility vary widely.

Side effects are common, especially early on. Around 60 to 70 percent of patients experience gastrointestinal symptoms, most often nausea (30 to 32 percent), diarrhea (18 to 23 percent), and vomiting (12 to 14 percent). These effects tend to be dose-related and often improve with slower dose escalation and time.

Semaglutide (Wegovy, Ozempic)

Third and fourth place are held by injectable semaglutide options (Wegovy, Ozempic), which can help you achieve around 15 percent weight loss when combined with healthy eating and activity changes.

Reference: Wilding JPH, et al. Once-Weekly Semaglutide in Adults with Overweight or Obesity. *N Engl J Med.* 2021;384:989-1002. doi:10.1056/NEJMoa2032183

Monthly costs for injectable semaglutide commonly range from $1,200 to $1,500 without insurance coverage. Some manufacturer-sponsored self-pay programs may reduce the price to about $499 per month, but these programs may change over time and are not guaranteed.

Side effects are similar to other GLP-1 receptor agonists. About 60 to 65 percent of patients report gastrointestinal symptoms, with nausea (44 percent), diarrhea (30 percent), and vomiting (24 percent) being the most common. As with tirzepatide, side effects often improve with gradual dose increases and supportive nutrition strategies.

Phentermine–Topiramate (Qsymia)

Fifth place is phentermine–topiramate (Qsymia), which can produce 9 to 10 percent weight loss.

Reference: Gadde KM, et al. Effects of low-dose, controlled-release, phentermine plus topiramate combination on weight and associated comorbidities in overweight and obese adults. *Lancet.* 2011;377(9774):1341-1352. doi:10.1016/S0140-6736(11)60205-5

Compared with injectable medications, Qsymia is generally more affordable. Without insurance, monthly costs average around $311, but savings programs and coupons can lower out-of-pocket expenses to roughly $79 to $98 per month for some patients.

Side effects occur in about 30 to 35 percent of users. The most common include dry mouth (21 percent), constipation (16 percent), and paresthesia or tingling sensations (14 percent). Because this medication contains a stimulant component, careful screening and monitoring are important.

Liraglutide (Saxenda, Victoza)

The sixth and seventh places are held by derivatives of liraglutide (Saxenda, Victoza), with results of around 8 percent weight loss over a year.

Reference: Pi-Sunyer X, et al. A Randomized, Controlled Trial of 3.0 mg of Liraglutide in Weight Management. *N Engl J Med.* 2015;373:11-22. doi:10.1056/NEJMoa1411892

Retail prices for liraglutide hover around $1,350 per month. However, for patients with insurance coverage or access to manufacturer savings programs, monthly costs may drop significantly, in some cases as low as $25 per month for up to 12 months.

Side effects are common and largely gastrointestinal. About 60 percent of patients report symptoms, most often nausea (40 percent), diarrhea (21 percent), and vomiting (16 percent). Because liraglutide is a daily injection, tolerability and adherence can be limiting factors for some individuals.

Oral Semaglutide (Rybelsus)

Eighth place is the first oral Semaglutide option (Rybelsus), offering 5 to 10 percent weight loss.

Reference: Davies M, et al. Oral semaglutide 50 mg for the treatment of obesity: the OASIS 1 trial. *Lancet.* 2023;402(10399):203-213. doi:10.1016/S0140-6736(23)01110-9

List prices for oral semaglutide typically range from about $998 to $1,100 per month. With insurance coverage and manufacturer savings programs, some patients may pay as little as $10 per month, though eligibility requirements apply.

Side effects are somewhat less frequent than injectable GLP-1 options but still common. About 50 to 55 percent of patients report symptoms, most often nausea (20 percent), diarrhea (15 percent), and vomiting (9 percent). Strict dosing instructions, like taking the medication on an empty stomach, are important for effectiveness.

Exenatide (Byetta, Bydureon)

Ninth place is held by Exenatide (Byetta, Bydureon). This drug has similar weight-loss achievement as Rybelsus at 5 to 10 percent weight loss but ranks lower on this list due to the need for more frequent injections.

Reference: Buse JB, et al. Exenatide once weekly versus twice daily for the treatment of type 2 diabetes. *Ann Intern Med.* 2011;154(2):103-112. doi:10.7326/0003-4819-154-2-201101180-00300

A one-month supply of exenatide generally costs between $838 and $950, depending on the formulation and dose. Insurance coverage varies, and fewer savings programs are available compared with newer agents.

Between 45 to 50 percent of patients report side effects, most commonly nausea (34 percent), diarrhea (13 percent), and vomiting (10 percent). Injection-site reactions can also occur, particularly with extended-release formulations.

Naltrexone–Bupropion (Contrave)

The tenth and final drug on this list is naltrexone–bupropion (Contrave), which generally helps you lose about 5 to 8 percent total body weight loss.

Reference: Greenway FL, et al. Naltrexone/bupropion for weight management in overweight and obese adults. *Lancet.* 2010;376(9741):595-605. doi:10.1016/S0140-6736(10)60888-4

The list price for Contrave is around $625 per month. Manufacturer programs such as CurAccess may reduce the cost to approximately $99 per month, and coupons can sometimes lower prices to around $199.

Side effects occur in roughly 30 to 40 percent of patients. The most common include nausea (33 percent), constipation (19 percent), and headache (18 percent). Because this medication affects brain signaling, careful attention to mental health history is important when considering its use.

REMEMBER

The first runner-up (honorable mention) would be Trulicity (dulaglutide) at higher doses when taken with metformin for added metabolic improvements to achieve 2 to 6 percent weight loss.

Reference: Ludvik B, et al. Efficacy and Safety of Once-Weekly Dulaglutide 3.0 mg and 4.5 mg Versus 1.5 mg in Type 2 Diabetes in the AWARD-11 Trial. *Diabetes Care.* 2021;44(3):765-773. doi:10.2337/dc20-1473

Monthly costs typically range from $887 to $1,400, depending on insurance coverage and assistance programs. Some patients may qualify for manufacturer programs that reduce costs to as little as $25 for a set number of pens.

About 50 percent of patients report side effects, most commonly nausea (12 to 21 percent), diarrhea (9 to 13 percent), and abdominal pain (7 to 10 percent). These effects are usually mild to moderate and often improve over time.

Chapter **12**

Top Ten Studies That Can Inform Your Weight-Loss Journey

I f you're exploring weight-loss medications, you'll want to know about the landmark studies that are shaping what's possible today. While it is important to review studies that are current, such as five years old or less, there are bedrock principles of weight-loss care that you can learn from older studies, too.

First, you will review the papers that summarize this evidence. That's right, you're going to see the guidelines your medical teams use. One of the themes you have picked up along the way of reading this book is the high value and importance of making meaningful, sustainable changes in dietary habits, lifestyle management strategies, and engagement in mindfulness as well as behavioral health tools.

This chapter will walk you through the research that backs up these recommendations. Afterwards, you will dive into the evidence that supports, or refutes, the claims for some dietary supplements (like green tea extracts). You will then get into the nitty gritty of what the scientific literature say about these GLP-RAs in regard to efficacy and what can happen if you stop them. Finally, you will review the real evidence behind the most well-studied adjuncts or alternatives to weight-loss medications you can turn to if your weight-loss journey stalls- bariatric surgery.

By understanding these key takeaways, you can have more informed conversations with your team and feel confident about your next steps in managing your weight and health.

Reframing Obesity as a Chronic Disease That Deserves Structured Care

American Association of Clinical Endocrinologists and American College of Endocrinology Clinical Practice Guidelines

Goal: To explain how experts define obesity as a chronic disease and use this framework to guide treatment decisions

Key takeaways: These guidelines underscore that obesity isn't simply about losing pounds; it's about reducing disease risk and improving overall health. By taking a personalized, staged, and evidence-based approach, they emphasize realistic early goals and offer a clear roadmap — from lifestyle changes to medications and surgery — for achieving lasting health benefits.

The American Association of Clinical Endocrinologists (AACE) and the American College of Endocrinology (ACE) Comprehensive Clinical Practice Guidelines for Medical Care of Patients with Obesity (https://pubmed.ncbi.nlm.nih. gov/27219496/) from 2016 presented a fundamental shift in the management of adults with obesity. The AACE and ACE are leading professional organizations representing physicians and experts who specialize in hormone, metabolic, and obesity-related diseases. Their joint clinical practice guidelines are widely used by healthcare teams to standardize high-quality, evidence-based obesity care.

Ahead of its time, this guideline describes obesity as a chronic, adiposity-based disease and recommends a structured, complication-centered approach to care. Treatment is personalized based on both BMI and the presence or severity of health complications, using a staged framework (overweight stage 0, obesity stage 1, obesity stage 2) to guide intervention intensity. They emphasize early weight loss — targeting at least 2.5 percent body weight reduction within the first month — as a predictor of long-term success, and recommend at least 5 percent, or ideally 10 percent, weight loss to improve health outcomes in many patients. Core treatment includes high-intensity lifestyle therapy, with early escalation to anti-obesity medications and consideration of bariatric surgery for appropriate patients.

Reference: Garvey WT, Mechanick JI, Brett EM, Garber AJ, Hurley DL, Jastreboff AM, Nadolsky K, Pessah-Pollack R, Plodkowski R; Reviewers of the AACE/ACE Obesity Clinical Practice Guidelines. AMERICAN ASSOCIATION OF CLINICAL ENDOCRINOLOGISTS AND AMERICAN COLLEGE OF ENDOCRINOLOGY COMPRE-HENSIVE CLINICAL PRACTICE GUIDELINES FOR MEDICAL CARE OF PATIENTS WITH OBESITY. *Endocr Pract.* 2016 Jul;22 Suppl 3:1-203. doi: 10.4158/EP161365. GL. Epub 2016 May 24. PMID: 27219496.

When Bariatric Surgery Becomes a Treatment, Not a Last Resort

Goal: To clarify when bariatric surgery should be considered and who may benefit based on health risk rather than body size alone

Key takeaways: These updated guidelines reflect today's advanced surgical techniques and a growing understanding of obesity as a treatable disease not just a number on the scale. By lowering BMI thresholds and accounting for metabolic risk profiles (including by ethnicity), the ASMBS and IFSO are helping more patients access a proven, safe, and effective treatment option that can improve long-term health and quality of life.

These guidelines were developed by the American Society for Metabolic and Bariatric Surgery (ASMBS) and the International Federation for the Surgery of Obesity and Metabolic Disorders (IFSO), two globally recognized organizations that set standards for safe, effective surgical treatment of obesity and metabolic disease.

This joint ASMBS and IFSO guideline (https://pubmed.ncbi.nlm.nih.gov/ 36336720/) details when metabolic and bariatric surgery should be considered. Those guidelines expand the 1991 NIH criteria by recommending surgery for any adult with a body mass index (BMI) equal to or greater than 35, regardless of whether obesity-related conditions are present. They also advise considering surgery for those with a BMI between 30 and 34.9 if they have metabolic disease, such as type 2 diabetes or hypertension. For Asian individuals, who face higher metabolic risks at lower BMIs, surgery is suggested starting at BMI equal to or greater than 27.5. The guidelines also encourage considering surgery for appro-priately selected children and adolescents with severe obesity.

Reference: Eisenberg D, Shikora SA, Aarts E, Aminian A, Angrisani L, Cohen RV, de Luca M, Faria SL, Goodpaster KPS, Haddad A, Himpens JM, Kow L, Kurian M, Loi K, Mahawar K, Nimeri A, O'Kane M, Papasavas PK, Ponce J, Pratt JSA, Rogers AM, Steele KE, Suter M, Kothari SN. 2022 American Society of Metabolic and Bariatric Surgery (ASMBS) and International Federation for the Surgery of Obesity and Metabolic Disorders (IFSO) Indications for Metabolic and Bariatric Surgery. *Obes Surg.* 2023 Jan;33(1):3-14. doi: 10.1007/s11695-022-06332-1. Erratum in: *Obes Surg.* 2023 Jan;33(1):15-16. doi: 10.1007/s11695-022-06369-2. PMID: 36336720; PMCID: PMC9834364.

Treating Childhood Obesity Early to Change Lifelong Health Trajectories

American Academy of Pediatrics Clinical Practice Guideline

The American Academy of Pediatrics (AAP) is the primary professional organization guiding pediatric medical care in the United States. Its clinical practice guidelines strongly influence how pediatricians diagnose, counsel, and treat children with obesity across diverse healthcare settings.

Goal: To show why early treatment of childhood obesity improves long-term health outcomes

Key takeaways: These guidelines mark a significant shift in pediatric obesity care, advocating for early, proactive, and holistic treatment rather than delayed action. By recognizing obesity's complex roots and supporting personalized, comprehensive interventions, the AAP aims to offer better health outcomes for millions of children who previously received minimal or ineffective treatment.

The Clinical Practice Guideline for the Evaluation and Treatment of Children and Adolescents With Obesity was published by the American Academy of Pediatrics (AAP) in 2023 (https://pubmed.ncbi.nlm.nih.gov/36622115/). This was the AAP's first comprehensive guideline in nearly 15 years for evaluating and treating children and adolescents (ages 2 to 18) with obesity, recognizing it as a chronic disease influenced by biological, socioeconomic, and environmental factors, not just lifestyle alone.

The guideline discards the outdated "watchful waiting" approach, instead calling for immediate, evidence-based interventions, including family-centered behavioral change, consideration of medication (for ages 12 and up), and even bariatric surgery (for those 13 and up), when appropriate. It emphasizes that treatment plans should be tailored to each child's unique context, including family dynamics, access to healthy food and activity, availability of support long-term, and sustainable behavior changes.

Reference: Hampl SE, Hassink SG, Skinner AC, Armstrong SC, Barlow SE, Bolling CF, Avila Edwards KC, Eneli I, Hamre R, Joseph MM, Lunsford D, Mendonca E, Michalsky MP, Mirza N, Ochoa ER, Sharifi M, Staiano AE, Weedn AE, Flinn SK, Lindros J, Okechukwu K. Clinical Practice Guideline for the Evaluation and Treatment of Children and Adolescents with Obesity. *Pediatrics*. 2023 Feb 1;151(2):e2022060640. doi: 10.1542/peds.2022-060640. Erratum in: Pediatrics. 2024 Jan 1;153(1):e2023064612. doi: 10.1542/peds.2023-064612. PMID: 36622115.

Why the Best Diet Is the One You Can Stick With

A TO Z Comparative Weight Loss Study

Goal: To help you choose a diet you can follow long term rather than chasing the latest trend

Key takeaways: The A to Z Comparative Weight Loss Study challenged the idea that one popular diet is universally superior for everyone. While Atkins produced the largest average weight loss, the differences between diets were not dramatic, and individual success depended more on sticking to the plan than on which diet it was. This means that for many people, the best diet is the one they can follow long-term, emphasizing sustainability and personal preference over chasing the latest trend. It also set the stage for later research focusing less on diet "brand names" and more on behavioral strategies, adherence, and individual metabolic responses.

The A to Z Study (https://pubmed.ncbi.nlm.nih.gov/17341711/) was a one-year randomized trial that compared four popular diet plans — Atkins, Zone, Ornish, and LEARN — among overweight and obese premenopausal women. Results showed that participants following the low-carbohydrate Atkins diet lost the most weight, averaging around 10 pounds at 12 months, while the other groups (Zone, Ornish, LEARN) experienced more modest losses. The study highlighted that diet adherence was a key factor, with those who stuck most closely to their assigned diet achieving the greatest weight loss, regardless of diet type.

Reference: Gardner CD, Kiazand A, Alhassan S, Kim S, Stafford RS, Balise RR, Kraemer HC, King AC. Comparison of the Atkins, Zone, Ornish, and LEARN Diets for Change in Weight and Related Risk Factors among Overweight Premenopausal Women: The A TO Z Weight Loss Study: A Randomized Trial. *JAMA*. 2007 Mar 7;297(9):969-77. doi: 10.1001/jama.297.9.969. Erratum in: JAMA. 2007 Jul 11;298(2):178. PMID: 17341711.

The Power and Limits of Intensive Lifestyle Change in Type 2 Diabetes

Goal: To explain what intensive lifestyle change can realistically achieve for weight, fitness, and overall health

Key takeaways: The intensive lifestyle intervention (ILI) didn't lower heart attack or stroke rates. However, many other health benefits including improved physical fitness, metabolism, mood, and quality of life were captured. These findings demonstrate that structured, comprehensive lifestyle change remains foundational in managing type 2 diabetes. Importantly, a recent analysis of Look AHEAD data found that combining at least 7 percent weight loss with high physical activity levels was associated with a remarkable 61 percent reduction in cardiovascular events, highlighting the powerful synergy of weight loss plus exercise.

The Look AHEAD study (https://pubmed.ncbi.nlm.nih.gov/20876408/) was a large, long-term randomized controlled trial involving over 5,000 overweight or obese adults with type 2 diabetes. It compared an intensive lifestyle intervention (ILI), which included structured diet, physical activity, and behavioral support. This treatment group was then compared to subjects who experienced standard diabetes support and education (DSE) over nearly ten years. The ILI group achieved significant weight loss (8.6 percent after one year and 6.2 percent at four years), along with improved fitness, better blood glucose control, lower blood pressure, fewer sleep apnea symptoms, and enhanced quality of life, but the intervention initially did not reduce the rate of major cardiovascular events like heart attacks or strokes.

Reference: Look AHEAD Research Group; Wing RR. Long-Term Effects of a Lifestyle Intervention on Weight and Cardiovascular Risk Factors in Individuals with Type 2 Diabetes Mellitus: Four-Year Results of the Look AHEAD Trial. *Arch Intern Med*. 2010 Sep 27;170(17):1566-75. doi: 10.1001/archinternmed.2010.334. PMID: 20876408; PMCID: PMC3084497.

Making Behavioral Therapy for Obesity Work in Real-World Primary Care

Goal: To demonstrate how structured behavioral therapy for obesity can be delivered effectively in primary care settings

Key takeaways: The MODEL–IBT Program bridges a major gap in obesity care by showing that a structured, practical behavioral health approach to enhance the weight-loss journey can be easily implemented in a primary care clinic. This is valuable considering that the primary care clinic is where most people receive their healthcare and obesity medicine management. The MODEL–IBT Program's success in delivering sustainable, moderate weight loss demonstrates the power of consistent, behavior-focused counseling, making obesity treatment more accessible, effective, and scalable across diverse healthcare settings.

The MODEL–IBT Program (`https://pubmed.ncbi.nlm.nih.gov/31544345/`) was developed to give primary care providers a practical, evidence-based protocol for delivering intensive behavioral therapy (IBT) for obesity, building on the Centers for Medicare & Medicaid Services' (CMS) coverage guidelines. It consists of twenty-one counseling visits over one year — weekly for the first month, biweekly through six months, and then monthly through one year. In a randomized trial using this schedule, patients achieved an average 6.1 percent weight loss at twelve months, with 44 percent of participants losing at least 5 percent of their baseline weight.

Reference: Wadden TA, Tsai AG, Tronieri JS. A Protocol to Deliver Intensive Behavioral Therapy (IBT) for Obesity in Primary Care Settings: The MODEL–IBT Program. *Obesity (Silver Spring)*. 2019 Oct;27(10):1562-1566. doi: 10.1002/oby.22594. PMID: 31544345; PMCID: PMC6786257.

Separating Hype from Evidence in Weight-Loss Supplements

Goal: To help you evaluate weight-loss supplements using evidence instead of marketing claims

Key takeaways: This review underscores that while dietary supplements can offer small metabolic benefits, they are not substitutes for evidence-based prescription therapies like GLP-1 receptor agonists or bariatric surgery when significant weight loss is the goal. For patients drawn to "natural" options, it highlights the importance of realistic expectations, potential safety concerns, and the need for medical guidance. Ultimately, the evidence shows these products may play only a minor, supportive role in a comprehensive weight management plan.

This review (https://pmc.ncbi.nlm.nih.gov/articles/PMC9099655/) examined commonly used supplements marketed for weight loss, including caffeine, green tea extract, green coffee bean extract, choline, glucomannan, and capsaicinoids. It evaluated both their potential metabolic effects and safety profiles using available clinical and observational studies. Overall, most supplements showed modest effects on body weight, generally much smaller than those achieved with FDA-approved weight-loss medications. Some, like caffeine and green tea extract, demonstrated small increases in energy expenditure or fat oxidation, while glucomannan showed mild appetite suppression in some trials. Safety was generally acceptable at recommended doses, though certain products can interact with medications or cause gastrointestinal discomfort. The authors noted a lack of large, high-quality randomized controlled trials, making it difficult to draw strong conclusions about long-term efficacy or safety.

WARNING

Importantly, new research highlights the lack of regulation and potential safety concerns around these unproven options. If you're considering them, it's crucial to proceed with caution and consult a healthcare provider, especially since real, clinically validated medications offer more predictable, durable benefits for weight management.

Reference: Mah E, Chen O, Liska DJ, Blumberg JB. Dietary Supplements for Weight Management: A Narrative Review of Safety and Metabolic Health Benefits. *Nutrients.* 2022 Apr 24;14(9):1787. doi: 10.3390/nu14091787. PMID: 35565754; PMCID: PMC9099655.

Choosing between Leading Medications Using Head-to-Head Evidence

SURMOUNT 5 Trial

Goal: To compare two leading weight-loss medications using direct clinical evidence

Key takeaways: This study gives you clear, head-to-head evidence that tirzepatide produces significantly greater weight loss than semaglutide in adults with obesity who do not have diabetes. That matters because, until now, most studies compared these drugs only to placebo. That means patients and clinicians were unsure which might be more effective when choosing between them. This trial helps guide real-world treatment decisions, especially for people who have tried other medications with limited success or want the most effective option supported by direct comparative data. It also reinforces the role of GLP-1/GIP combination drugs like tirzepatide as a leading next-step therapy for substantial, sustainable weight loss.

In this pivotal Phase 3b randomized trial called "SURMOUNT-5" (https://pubmed.ncbi.nlm.nih.gov/40353578/), adults with obesity but no type 2 diabetes were assigned to receive weekly injections of either tirzepatide (10 to 15 mg) or semaglutide (1.7 to 2.4 mg) for 72 weeks. At the end of the study period, the tirzepatide group achieved a mean body weight reduction of approximately 20.2 percent, compared to about 13.7 percent in the semaglutide group, a statistically significant difference. Participants using tirzepatide also experienced a greater decrease in waist circumference by more than 5 centimeters. Overall, the findings demonstrate that tirzepatide offers superior weight-loss outcomes compared to semaglutide in this population.

Reference: Aronne LJ, Horn DB, le Roux CW, Ho W, Falcon BL, Gomez Valderas E, Das S, Lee CJ, Glass LC, Senyucel C, Dunn JP; SURMOUNT-5 Trial Investigators. Tirzepatide as Compared with Semaglutide for the Treatment of Obesity. *N Engl J Med.* 2025 Jul 3;393(1):26-36. doi: 10.1056/NEJMoa2416394. Epub 2025 May 11. PMID: 40353578.

What Happens When Weight-Loss Medication Is Stopped

Semaglutide Treatment Effect in People with Obesity Trial Extension

Goal: To explain what typically happens when weight-loss medication is stopped

Key takeaways: This extension study illustrates the chronic nature of obesity and emphasizes that discontinuing semaglutide and stopping your supportive lifestyle interventions can lead to significant weight regain and loss of initial health benefits. The findings highlight the importance of ongoing treatment and follow-up to sustain weight loss and its related health improvements.

The STEP-1 Extension Study (https://pubmed.ncbi.nlm.nih.gov/35441470/) was a part of the STEP clinical trial series on semaglutide for weight management of adults without type 2 diabetes. After completing sixty-eight weeks of once-weekly 2.4 mg semaglutide treatment, participants entered an off-treatment follow-up period lasting roughly fifty-two weeks. During this withdrawal phase, they regained approximately 11.6 percentage points of the weight they had previously lost, resulting in a net weight loss of about 5.6 percent from baseline, down from an initial 17.3 percent loss Corresponding cardiometabolic benefits (like improvements in blood pressure, lipids, and glucose control) largely reverted toward baseline as well.

Reference: Wilding JPH, Batterham RL, Davies M, Van Gaal LF, Kandler K, Konakli K, Lingvay I, McGowan BM, Oral TK, Rosenstock J, Wadden TA, Wharton S, Yokote K, Kushner RF; STEP 1 Study Group. Weight Regain and Cardiometabolic Effects after Withdrawal of Semaglutide: The STEP 1 Trial Extension. *Diabetes Obes Metab.* 2022 Aug;24(8):1553-1564. doi: 10.1111/dom.14725. Epub 2022 May 19. PMID: 35441470; PMCID: PMC9542252.

Medications versus Surgery: Understanding the Tradeoffs for Long-Term Weight Loss

Systematic Review and Meta Analysis of GLP 1 Receptor Agonists versus Bariatric Surgery

Goal: To help you compare long-term weight-loss outcomes from medications versus surgery

Key takeaways: This study highlights that, while GLP-1 medications are a valuable, less invasive option for weight management, bariatric surgery remains the most powerful intervention for substantial and sustained weight loss in adults with obesity. For some patients, especially those with severe obesity or obesity-related complications, these bariatric surgery results can inform shared decision-making about treatment pathways. In short, if long-term, large-scale weight loss is the goal, current evidence strongly favors surgery, though individual risk tolerance, health status, and treatment preferences remain key factors.

The systematic review and meta-analysis compared weight-loss outcomes from GLP-1 receptor agonists (GLP-RAs) like semaglutide and liraglutide with various bariatric surgeries, including gastric bypass and sleeve gastrectomy (https://pubmed.ncbi.nlm.nih.gov/36321278/). Across multiple studies, bariatric surgery produced significantly greater total body weight loss than GLP-1 RAs, with a mean difference of about -22.68 kg and a BMI reduction of -8.18 in favor of surgery. The analysis also found that surgery was more effective at achieving clinically meaningful weight-loss thresholds (equal or greater than 20 percent of body weight). While GLP-1 RAs did improve weight and metabolic parameters, their effects were smaller and less durable than those seen after surgery. The study noted that surgical patients often maintained their weight loss for years, whereas weight regain after medication discontinuation was common. Safety profiles differed — surgery carried higher upfront procedural risks, while GLP-1 RAs had mainly gastrointestinal side effects.

Reference: Sarma S, Palcu P. Weight Loss between Glucagon-Like Peptide-1 Receptor Agonists and Bariatric Surgery in Adults with Obesity: A Systematic Review and Meta-Analysis. *Obesity (Silver Spring)*. 2022 Nov;30(11):2111–2121. doi: 10.1002/oby.23563. PMID: 36321278.

Chapter **13**

Top Ten Alternatives to Weight-Loss Medicines

When weight-loss medications don't give you the full results you hoped for, it's easy to feel stuck. The truth is that there are many powerful alternatives worth exploring. Some of the most effective options are procedure-based, like bariatric surgery and endoscopic bariatric procedures, which can create major, long-lasting changes (see Chapter 10 for more on weight-loss surgery). These permanent interventions alter appetite, metabolism, and overall health.

Others alternatives are rooted in lifestyle. Behavioral strategies help you untangle emotional eating and build positive habits you can maintain, and exercise and diet play huge roles, too. Activity not only burns calories, but also boosts your mood, and even improves your insulin sensitivity. And when it comes to what you eat, two paths consistently rise to the top: the Mediterranean diet and high-protein, moderate-carbohydrate diets that keep you full and protect your muscle.

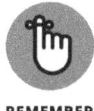

REMEMBER

None of these strategies are magic on their own, but together they form a toolbox of options that can move the needle when medications fall short. Think of this chapter as your roadmap to the top ten evidence-backed alternatives to weight-loss drugs. It's all about finding what works for your body, your lifestyle, and your long-term health.

Bariatric Surgery

Bariatric surgery is the most effective non-pharmacologic treatment we have for severe obesity with long-term average total body weight loss of about 20 to 30 percent, depending on the procedure. In a large, long-term study comparing surgery to medical and lifestyle care, people who had bariatric surgery maintained about 19 to 20 percent weight loss at seven to twelve years, versus 8 to 11 percent in those treated with lifestyle and medications alone. Five-year data show around 22 to 26 percent TBWL for Roux-en-Y Gastric Bypass and 16 to 23 percent TBWL for sleeve gastrectomy. Some of the newer or more aggressive procedures, like duodenal switch variants, can reach 30 to 35 percent TBWL at one to two years.

Beyond the scale, surgery also improves type 2 diabetes, hypertension, sleep apnea, and MASLD/NAFLD in a large share of patients. In short, bariatric surgery reliably delivers about one-quarter of total body weight lost and kept off long-term for many patients, which is far more than any lifestyle program or supplement can offer. See Chapter 10 more on these surgery types.

Endoscopic Bariatric Procedures

You might consider endoscopic bariatric therapies the "middle-ground" options that do not involve traditional surgery but still produce more weight loss than lifestyle change alone. Endoscopic Sleeve Gastroplasty (ESG) typically leads to about 13 to 20 percent total body weight loss at twelve months. In a recent study, ESG patients lost 13.6 percent TBWL at one year versus 0.8 percent in the lifestyle-only control group.

Intragastric balloon (IGB) therapy usually produces 10 to 15 percent TBWL at six to twelve months, and a recent review confirmed significantly greater excess-weight loss at six, nine, and twelve months compared with standard care. However, you must be aware that weight regain can occur after balloon removal, so long-term success depends heavily on ongoing your good habits including diet, activity, and behavioral support (see Chapter 5 for more on lifestyle changes). Overall, endoscopic procedures usually deliver about half to two-thirds of the weight loss of surgery with lower procedural risk, making them strong options for people who are not ready for or do not qualify for bariatric surgery. See Chapter 10 for more details on surgical weight-loss alternatives.

Behavioral Lifestyle Changes

Cognitive Behavioral Therapy (CBT) and structured behavioral programs typically lead to 5 to 8 percent total body weight loss when combined with diet and activity. CBT helps you to identify emotional triggers, reduce binge-eating behaviors, and change unhelpful thought patterns that derail your weight-loss journey. Studies show that adding CBT to standard diet programs improves weight loss by an additional 6.6 to 11 pounds (3 to 5 kg). Programs that include self-monitoring, goal setting, problem-solving, stimulus control (removing triggers), and regular follow-up produce the highest success rates. Acceptance and Commitment Therapy (ACT), mindfulness-based therapy, and motivational interviewing also show benefits, helping reduce emotional eating and improve long-term maintenance. If you engage in structured behavioral therapy during weight-loss attempts, you are twice as likely to maintain weight loss over two years compared with those who rely on diet alone.

TIP

CBT and behavioral strategies don't directly "burn calories," but they change the habits and thought patterns that make weight loss lasting. In addition, behavioral therapies consistently improve outcomes across all treatment types.

Exercise

Exercise alone produces modest but meaningful weight loss, typically 2 to 3 percent total body weight loss over six to twelve months when not combined with dietary changes. You might think of this as an option if you are active but not ready to commit to altered diet patterns. A large review of aerobic training showed an average loss of about 4.4 to 6.6 pounds (2.0 to 3.0 kg) and reductions in waist circumference even without calorie restriction. When people combine aerobic exercise with resistance training, studies show 3 to 5 percent TBWL, better fat loss, and better preservation of lean mass. High-intensity interval training (HIIT) can reduce BMI by about 1.3 points and body fat by 2 to 4 percent, even with minimal weekly time commitments.

These are important considerations if your free time to commit to a weight-loss program is limited throughout the week. Importantly, exercise dramatically increases the chances of keeping weight off. One long-term study showed that patients maintaining more than 200 minutes of exercise per week kept off 28.7 pounds (13 kg) more compared with those who did not. Consider making 200 minutes of aerobic exercise per week your starting goal. Exercise also improves blood sugar, lowers blood pressure, and reduces liver fat independent of weight loss.

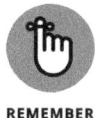

REMEMBER Exercise alone may give you modest weight loss, but when paired with diet or medication, it significantly boosts your results and protects your long-term weight-loss success.

Mediterranean Diet

The Mediterranean diet is an eating pattern built around vegetables, fruits, whole grains, beans, nuts, olive oil, and lean proteins like fish and poultry, with minimal processed foods and sweets. This diet option may be the smartest choice you make in your journey. The Mediterranean diet has some of the strongest evidence for steady, sustainable weight loss and major improvements in overall metabolic health, and it's not even built on calorie restrictions. In one large trial, people following this way of eating lost 9.7 to 22.3 pounds (4.4 to 10.1 kg) over a year. Other research shows that the Mediterranean diet leads to more long-term weight loss than low-fat diets. It has also been shown to reduce major cardiovascular events by about 30 percent, which makes it one of the most heart-protective eating patterns available. Overall, the Mediterranean diet stands out as one of the safest, most effective approaches for both weight control and long-term metabolic benefits. See Chapter 7 for more information on how this diet complements your nutrient needs, and see Chapter 9 for more details about this particular diet.

High-Protein, Moderate-Carbohydrate Diet

A high-protein, moderate-carbohydrate (HPMC) diet is an eating pattern that increases your protein intake to about 25 to 30 percent of your daily **calories** while keeping carbohydrates at a steady, moderate level rather than very low. This usually means prioritizing foods like lean meats, fish, eggs, Greek yogurt, beans, and tofu. This allows you to include moderate portions of whole-grain carbs such as brown rice, quinoa, and fruits. Higher-protein, moderate-carbohydrate diets have solid evidence behind them, especially when it comes to improving fullness, increasing fat loss, and helping preserve muscle during weight reduction. In one large review of twenty-four trials, people eating a higher-protein diet lost about 1.7 pounds (0.79 kg) more over twelve weeks than those eating standard-protein diets. This approach also boasts improvements in triglycerides and blood pressure. You should be aware that the HPMC diet correlates with approximately 3 to 5 percent TBWL, which is less than the Mediterranean diet. This approach seems to work especially well if your body has insulin resistance or metabolic syndrome. Overall, higher-protein diets can offer you a practical, satisfying way to support steady weight loss while protecting your muscles and metabolic health.

Fiber Supplements

Fiber supplements can make weight loss easier because they help you feel full sooner and stay full longer, which naturally reduces how much you eat. In one study, people who drank a higher-protein, higher-fiber shake before meals lost 7.3 pounds (3.3 kg) in twelve weeks, compared with 4.0 pounds (1.8 kg) in the lower-fiber group. Another trial showed that fiber changes how your body digests food by slowing gastric emptying, lowering the "energy density" of your meals, and even feeding your gut bacteria. Fiber digestion can produce short-chain fatty acids, which support healthier blood sugar control and appetite signals. Mechanistically, fiber increases the thickness (viscosity) of food in the stomach and small intestine, which triggers stretch receptors and GLP-1–related satiety pathways, so you feel satisfied on fewer calories.

TECHNICAL STUFF

Different types of fiber work in different ways: wheat dextrin is a non-viscous, fermentable fiber that blends easily into foods and improves fullness with doses of 2 to 6 g per meal. Psyllium and methylcellulose are viscous fibers that thicken in the gut, helping slow digestion and stabilize blood sugar, which can prevent overeating later in the day. Pectin and guar gum, which is found in foods like apples, green beans, and sweet potatoes, are both viscous and fermentable, meaning they help with fullness immediately and improve gut health over time.

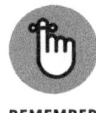

REMEMBER

A fiber-rich diet is lower in energy density, often has a lower fat content, and is richer in micronutrients, all of which have beneficial health effects. You should consider taking this small step to add fiber as an adjunct to your weight-loss journey.

Green Tea Extract (EGCG)

Green tea extract is one of the most well-studied supplements for weight loss, and while the results are modest, they are real. A large review of fifteen randomized trials found that people taking green tea catechins lost about **2.9 pounds** more than those taking a placebo over twelve weeks. Other studies show the best results when daily intake is over 300 mg of catechins.

TECHNICAL STUFF

A single green tea bag typically contains around 100 to 150 mg of polyphenols, with approximately 75 to 112 mg of epigallocatechin-3-gallate (EGCG), the main catechin.

Researchers think the effects come from a few different mechanisms: green tea can gently increase fat oxidation, slightly boost metabolic rate, and activate a hormone system that helps the body burn more stored fat. It may also help you to reduce LDL cholesterol and improve your post-meal blood sugar responses, which can indirectly support your weight management. You can expect 2.2 to 6.6 pounds (1 to 3 kg) of weight loss, which makes green tea extract a helpful add-on rather than a primary weight-loss strategy.

TIP

In terms of safety, green tea extract is generally well tolerated, but high doses can interact with stimulant medications and certain blood thinners. So, if you are going to take over 300 mg of catechins per day, then you should make sure to discuss this plan with your physician to reconcile your medication list. Very large amounts may stress the liver in sensitive individuals. When used at typical supplement doses and alongside other weight-loss medications, it is usually safe, but it's smart to check with your clinician if you have liver issues. Overall, green tea extract can give your weight-loss plan a gentle boost, especially when paired with healthy eating and regular movement. This supplement can support your weight-loss efforts, but it is best used alongside solid nutrition, movement, and lifestyle habits rather than as a stand-alone fix.

Probiotics

Probiotics are getting a lot of buzz for weight management, but the results so far are small and very mixed. The way probiotics seem to help is by shifting gut bacteria, lowering inflammation, and possibly reducing how much fat the body absorbs.

Some strains like *Lactobacillus gasseri* SBT2055 have been shown to help people lose about 1.4 percent of their body weight, which worked out to roughly 2.4 pounds (1.1 kg), along with a 1.5 percent drop in BMI and about a 1.8 percent reduction in waist size over twelve weeks. In another study, the same strain led to about an 8.5 percent decrease in visceral fat, which is the deeper, more harmful fat around the organs. A combination of other strains, including *Lactobacillus plantarum* KY1032, produced similar effects with meaningful reductions in body weight and waist measurements compared to placebo. Even with these positives, the overall weight loss is still pretty modest, only 2.2 to 6.6 pounds (1 to 3 kg) total.

REMEMBER

It appears that if you rely on this as the sole treatment in your weight loss, your results may fade when you stop taking the supplement. So while certain strains show real, measurable changes, they're still gentle nudges rather than major weight-loss tools. In the end, probiotics can support your efforts, but they're best used alongside your healthy eating and regular movement strategies, probiotics are not a replacement for healthy lifestyle.

Berberine

Berberine has gotten a lot of attention for weight loss — but the actual results are small, and the research is pretty inconsistent. Most studies show only about 4 pounds of total body weight loss, which is helpful but not dramatic. People also saw tiny changes in BMI and about a 1-centimeter drop in waist size. Berberine lowers fasting glucose and improves insulin sensitivity through activation of 5' adenosine monophosphate-activated protein kinase (AMPK), often described as the body's "metabolic master switch."

AMPK helps to control how much glucose your muscles take up and how much sugar your liver produces. In addition, berberine improves insulin sensitivity by increasing insulin receptor activity, making cells more responsive to the insulin your body already makes. On top of that, berberine reduces inflammation by lowering pro-inflammatory cytokines and oxidative stress, both of which play a role in insulin resistance.

When researchers looked at how people responded to berberine over time, they found that the longer someone took it, the more it helped with weight-related measures. Berberine led to small drops in BMI and a much bigger improvement in waist size as treatment continued. In simple terms, it didn't make a dramatic difference, but the benefits tended to grow the longer someone stayed on it.

While berberine can lower fasting glucose, improve insulin sensitivity, and reduce inflammation, the trials are usually short and small, so it's hard to know how reliable the results really are.

WARNING

Berberine also interacts with liver enzymes (like CYPs and P-glycoprotein), so it can change levels of other medications, including blood thinners, blood pressure meds, and some diabetes drugs. Combining berberine supplementation with GLP-RA treatments should only be done under medical supervision. Berberine may slightly support metabolic health and weight maintenance, but high-quality randomized clinical trials are still lacking. Berberine supplementation should be treated as an experimental add-on, not a proven cornerstone therapy.

Index

leptin receptor (LEPR) deficiency, 129

licensed therapists, 158

lifestyle-based care, 126

lifestyle coaching, 63

lifestyle factors
management, 155–156
and medication efficacy, 141–144

LillyDirect, 73

lipid panel
GLP medications, 54
monitoring, 109

liquid nutrition, 148

liraglutide, 145, 179
weight-loss outcomes, 192–193

liver and GLP medications, 54

liver function tests (LFTs), 109, 110

long-acting reversible contraceptives (LARCs), 123

long-term weight loss, 192
outcomes, 192–193

Look AHEAD study, 188

lorcaserin, 17

Lose It! (Snap It), 65, 99, 106

lunch, nutrient needs, 86

M

macronutrient, 78, 83
goals, 83

magnesium, 94
deficiency, 93

magnesium glycinate, 94

mail-order pharmacy, 68

malnutrition, 141

maridebart cafraglutide, 41

massage therapy, 159

mazdutide, 41

MC4R (melanocortin 4 receptor) gene, 140

meals, 85

Medicare coverage, 73

medication, weight-loss, 9, 177
challenges, 137
development process, 26–29
discontinuation of, 113–114, 191–192
FDA approved, 33–34
future of, 40
global trend, 21–22
ineffectiveness reasons, 138–139
liraglutide, 179
mismatch and ineffectiveness, 138
mobile apps for tracking, 98
need for, 47–48
oral semaglutide, 180
phentermine-topiramate, 179
safety standards, 15, 20
selection criteria, 39–40
semaglutide, 177, 178
vs surgery, 192
timeline, of weight-loss drugs, 19
tirzepatide, 177, 178

Medisafe, 98

Mediterranean diet, 154

melanocortin-4 receptor (MC4R) agonist, 130

menopause
and GLP-RAs impact, 124
and physical activity, 88

meridia. See sibutramine

metabolic dysfunction-associated steatotic liver disease (MASLD), 128, 134, 166, 167

metabolic enzyme inhibitors, 43

metabolic rate and cardiovascular exercise, 88

metabolic syndrome, 128

metabolism
and medication ineffectiveness, 138
in weight-loss, 140–141

metformin, 127
and naltrexone-bupropion, 181

microbiome-based therapies, 43

microdosing, 75

micronutrients, 78, 79, 94

mindful eating, 115
habits, 141

mindfulness, 115
online tools, 117
weight loss techniques, 116

Mindfulness-Based Eating Awareness Training (MB-EAT), 118

minerals, 78

mobile apps, weight management, 98–99

MODEL–IBT Program, 189

mood boost and cardiovascular exercise, 88

motivation, 22
reasons for weight loss, 22

MOTS-c, 160

Mounjaro. See tirzepatide

movement, 77

multivitamin, hair-focused, 93–94

muscle building, 90, 91

muscle loss, 83
and GLP-RA medications, deficiency of, 51

MyFitnessPal, 65, 99, 106

MyFitnessPal Premium, 99, 105

myrrh, 11

MyTherapy, 98

N

naltrexone-bupropion, 17, 32, 181

natural supplements, weight loss, 95–96

nausea
exenatide, 180

plateau and medication
ineffectiveness, 139

PlateMate, 105, 106

podcasts, 117

polycystic ovarian syndrome
and medication
ineffectiveness, 138

polygenetics, 140

polysomnography, 100

POMC deficiency, 130

postbiotics, 94

potassium, 78

Prader–Willi syndrome
(PWS), 129

ARD-101, 129

medications, 129

prebiotics, 94

pregnancy

and GLP-RAs impact, 122

weight-loss medications
during, 123

prescription, 67

access and availability, 69

convenience, 68

coordination with
care team, 69

cost, 69

filling weight-loss
medication, 67

legitimate pharmacies, 71

level of support, 69

mail-order pharmacy, 68

protocols, 73–76

red flags, safe, 71

regular clinic, 67

risks and side effects, 71

safety, 69

specialists, 67

telehealth services, 67

warning signs, 68

preservatives, in ultra-
processed foods, 81

pre-surgery assessment

age consideration,
165–166

checklist, 166–167

dependence on mobility
device, 165

eligibility criteria, 164–165

gait limitation, 165

vs GLP-RA medication, 168

nutrition instructions, 168

physical performance
testing, 165

and preparation, 166–168

primary care provider, 46

probiotics, 94, 95

processed foods, 80

progesterone, 124

proopiomelanocortin (POMC)
deficiency, 129

proprotein convertase subtilisin/
kexin type 1 (PCSK1)
deficiency, 129

protein, 78

daily targets, 83–84

intake, 154

options, 79

priorities, 79

rich diet, 84–85

supplementation, 88

Q

Qsymia. *See*
phentermine-topiramate

R

rainbow pill, 14

red light therapy, 161

reflux, GLP-related side
effects, 80

Registered Dietitian (RD), 46, 64

reliably, wearables, 102

resistance training, geriatric
patients, 132

retatrutide, 41

rifampin and medication
ineffectiveness, 139

Ro, 56, 57

Roman physicians, on
weight loss, 10

Roux-en-Y Gastric Bypass
(RYGB), 169

rowing, as fitness activity, 88

Rybelsus. *See* oral semaglutide;
semaglutide

RYGB. *See* Roux-en-Y Gastric
Bypass (RYGB)

S

safety standard, medications

in earlier decades, 15

early 20th century, 21

late 19th century, 21

tests and screening, 54–56

saffron, 11

for flavor, 85

sarcopenia, 131

Saxenda. *See* liraglutide

scammony, 10

SCOUT trial (Sibutramine
Cardiovascular OUTcomes
Trial), 16

screenings, for GLP
medications, 55–56.
See also laboratory tests

self-monitoring devices.
See wearable technologies

semaglutide, 50, 124,
145, 178, 191

discontinuation of, 191

vs endoscopic sleeve
gastroplasty, 174

oral, 180

STEP clinical trial series on, 191

weight-loss outcomes, 192–193

and weight regain, 191

serotonin, 94

vitamin, 78
  B12, 94
    abnormal level, 111
    deficiency, 93
    and GLP medications, 55
    and GLP-RA medications,
      deficiency of, 50
    monitoring, 109
  D, 94
    deficiency, 93
    and GLP medications, 55
    and GLP-RA medications,
      deficiency of, 51, 52
  K2, 94
vomiting
  exenatide, 180
  and GLP-RAs side
    effects, 146
  liraglutide, 179
  oral semaglutide side
    effects, 180
  semaglutide side
    effects, 178

W

walking, as fitness activity, 88
water, 143
wearable technologies
  Apple Watch, 99, 101
  calorie tracking and, 98
  continuous glucose monitors
    (CGM), 103
  Fitbit, 99, 101, 102
  Garmin, 99, 101
  Hexoskin, 102
  Oura Ring, 101, 102
  reliably, 102
  step-count wearables, 102
  vital-sign monitoring
    patches, 103
  WHOOP, 99
Wegovy, 127.
    See also semaglutide
weight regain
  after medication
    discontinuation, 53, 193

AI tools, prevention
    strategies, 114
  fear and anxiety of, 117–118
  prevention, 114
Weight Watchers (WW), 99
whole foods, 79
Whole Health Rx, 56, 57
WHOOP, 99
women's health and GLP-RAs
    impact, 122

X

Xenical. *See* orlistat

Y

yoga, 159

Z

Zepbound. *See* tirzepatide
Zofran, 139
Zone diet plan, 187

About the Authors

Patrick T. Reeves, MD, is quadruple board certified in Obesity Medicine, Pediatric Gastroenterology, General Pediatrics, and Clinical Informatics. He is an established clinician–scientist with extensive experience caring for both children and adults with medical complexity, including patients with rare and chronic gastrointestinal disorders. Dr. Reeves is an associate professor of Pediatrics at the Joe R. and Teresa Lozano Long School of Medicine at UT Health San Antonio and at the Uniformed Services University of the Health Sciences in Bethesda, Maryland. He also serves as an associate professor of Military Medicine at the Texas A&M University Health Science Center in College Station, Texas. Over the past decade, Dr. Reeves' research has focused on the intersection of patient education, chronic disease management, and care delivery for children and young adults with medical complexity. He is the founder and CEO of Wild Child Medicine, PLLC, a consulting firm dedicated to improving care for patients with complex medical needs. Dr. Reeves has pioneered an innovative mobile health technology known as *Clinical Action Plans*, which provide automated clinical decision support for medical teams while also serving as low–health-literacy, family-centered care plans to support home management of chronic conditions.

Tania Elliott, MD, is a board-certified internist and allergist with expertise in immunology, environmental health, and chronic inflammatory disease. She is widely recognized for translating complex medical science into practical, patient-centered guidance. Dr. Elliott completed medical school at Jefferson Medical College, residency training at Mount Sinai Medical Center, and fellowship training in allergy and immunology at NYU Winthrop Hospital. She has held academic appointments and currently serves on the Board of Regents for the American College of Allergy, Asthma, and Immunology. Dr. Elliott is the founder of Tania Elliott MD, a medical practice and educational platform dedicated to immune health. Through her clinical work, writing, and public education, she is committed to improving.

Dedication

This book is dedicated to our families, whose love, patience, and unwavering support made this work possible. You are our foundation, our inspiration, and the reason we strive to make a difference.

Author's Acknowledgments

Patrick Reeves, MD: I am deeply grateful to Dr. Joseph May for his unwavering support, mentorship, and encouragement throughout my journey to becoming an obesity medicine specialist. His belief in the importance of compassionate, evidence-based obesity care and his generous guidance helped shape both my professional path and the work presented in this book. I also deeply appreciate the support I received from the Wiley Publishing team during this process. I would like to extend special thanks to my outstanding Development Editor, Jennifer Connolly. Her knowledge of the Dummies format and her patient guidance helped me navigate each step of the process.

Publisher's Acknowledgments

Senior Acquisitions Editor: Tracy Boggier

Development Editor: Jennifer Connolly

Copy Editor: Jennifer Connolly

Editorial Assistant: Shannon Kucaj

Senior Managing Editor: Kristie Pyles

Production Editor: Bharaneedharan Murthy

Cover Image: © Eduardo Monroy/Shutterstock